The Human Body User Manual

The Human Body User Manual

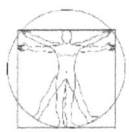

A Guide to Nature's Most Complex Engineering

Michael Wisdom

The information in this book is not intended to replace the advice of the reader's own physician or other medical professional. You should consult a medical professional in matters relating to health, especially if you have existing medical conditions, and before starting, stopping, or changing the dose of any medication you are taking. Individual readers are solely responsible for their own health-care decisions. The author and the publisher do not accept responsibility for any adverse effects individuals may claim to experience, whether directly or indirectly, from the information contained in this book.

All rights reserved. No part of this publication may be reproduced, stored in a retrieval system, or transmitted in any form or by any means—electronic, mechanical, photocopying, recording, or otherwise—without the prior written permission of the publisher, except for brief quotations used in reviews or scholarly works.

ISBN: 979-8-9931101-0-3
Library of Congress Control Number: 2025919920

All rights reserved. Printed in the United States of America
First Edition

Copyright © 2025 by Michael Wisdom
Windermere, FL

Published by Dictum Factum Press

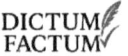

Dedication

To my wife, my partner in every adventure, and my daughter, the brightest spark of my imagination – this book is for you both.

Table of Contents

Part 1 – Orientation

1. Welcome to Your Human Body - 7

2. Specifications & Design Overview - 15

3. Safety Warnings & Operating Limits - 25

Part 2 – Core Systems & How They Work

4. The Frame: Skeletal System - 37

5. The Engine: Muscular System - 47

6. The Wiring: Nervous System - 57

7. The Power Supply: Cardiovascular System - 67

8. The Cooling & Waste Removal Systems: Respiratory & Excretory Systems - 77

9. The Control Panel: Endocrine & Immune Systems - 87

Part 3 – Maintenance & Upgrades

10. Fueling the Machine: Nutrition Basics - 99

11. Performance Upgrades: Exercise & Training - 109

12. Recovery Mode: Rest, Sleep, and Regeneration - 119

13. Routine Service Schedule - 127

Part 4 – Troubleshooting & Repairs

14. Warning Lights: Symptoms You Shouldn't Ignore - 137

15. Common Breakdowns & Fixes - 147

16. Software Errors: Mental & Emotional Health - 159

17. Emergency Repairs: What to Do When Things Go Wrong - 169

Part 5 – Optimization & Longevity

18. Performance Tuning: Lifestyle Habits for Longevity -181

19. Performance Tracking: Metrics That Matter - 191

20. Extending the Warranty: Preventive Care & Medical Advances - 199

Part 6 – Beyond Standard Use

21. Operating in Extreme Conditions - 209

22. Warranty & Service Life - 217

Epilogue – The Operator's Responsibility

Introduction

Why This Manual Exists

For years, I've had the privilege of working with clients across the spectrum — from individuals striving to feel stronger in daily life to executives at some of the top organizations in America who wanted to bring health and vitality into their high-pressure careers. In personal training, corporate wellness programs, and performance coaching, one theme kept surfacing: **people don't truly understand the machine they live in every day.**

It became almost a running joke. Someone would come into a session holding their brand-new iPhone or talking about their high-performance car, and they'd proudly share how they were learning all the hidden features by reading the manual or watching tutorials. They'd invest hours to unlock every capability of their newest piece of technology.

And yet — ask that same person a basic question about their body, and they'd shrug.

- Why is it important to learn how we should breathe during exercise?
- What makes your muscles stronger, or weaker?
- Why do you feel exhausted after certain meals but sharp after others?

Blank stares. Nervous laughter. Then the line I heard more times than I can count:
"Wouldn't it be nice if our bodies came with a user manual?"

That recurring comment stuck with me. Because the truth is, our bodies are **the most complex and advanced piece of engineering any of us will ever own.** No car, no phone, no piece of software comes close. Your body repairs itself, adapts to new stress, learns and rewires, cools and heats, filters and defends, and can perform brilliantly for decades. And yet most of us treat it like a black box — we push buttons, hope for the best, and deal with breakdowns only after they arrive.

This book was born out of that realization. If people will spend time learning their smartphone manual, why shouldn't they have one for the extraordinary system they already own? A guide not written for scientists, but for everyday operators. A reference you can return to again and again to understand the basics, troubleshoot the warning lights, and unlock your body's full performance potential.

That's what this book is: **your user manual.** Clear, practical, and written for the most important machine you'll ever operate.

Part 1

Orientation

Chapter 1

Welcome to Your Human Body

Why This Is the Most Advanced Piece of Engineering You'll Ever Own

Take a deep breath. Feel your chest rise, your ribs expand, your lungs stretch like finely tuned bellows. Without conscious effort, oxygen rushes in, carbon dioxide rushes out, and trillions of cells quietly hum with life. In that single breath, you've just witnessed one of the greatest feats of engineering in the known universe: **your body**.

We often marvel at the precision of supercomputers, the complexity of space shuttles, or the ingenuity behind skyscrapers. But none of these compare to the elegant, self-repairing, energy-conserving, multitasking marvel you live inside every single day.

Think about it:

- **Processing power:** Your brain, weighing just three pounds, contains about 86 billion neurons and more connections than there are stars in the Milky Way. No human-made machine even comes close.
- **Efficiency:** Your heart beats roughly 100,000 times a day without requiring replacement parts. Most pumps would wear out in a fraction of that time.
- **Durability:** Bones are stronger than concrete, yet lighter than steel. They're constantly breaking down and rebuilding themselves, upgrading as you age and adapt.
- **Self-repairing:** Scratch your skin, and in days it heals. Break a bone, and it fuses back together. Most machines, once broken, stay broken unless someone fixes them. Your body does it on its own.
- **Fuel flexibility:** While your car sputters without the exact grade of gasoline, your body can run on an astonishing variety of fuels — proteins, fats, carbohydrates — and still adapt, balance, and thrive.

- **Miniaturization:** Each of your cells is a microfactory, with power plants (mitochondria), recycling centers (lysosomes), highways (microtubules), and communication systems (receptors and ion channels).

It's not just advanced engineering — it's **living engineering**. Unlike any invention we've created, your body grows, adapts, learns, and upgrades itself.

And yet, most people walk around with only a vague understanding of how this system works. We've been given the most sophisticated device in history... but **no one handed us the instruction manual at birth**.

This book is meant to fix that.

Why a Manual?

Imagine buying the world's most advanced sports car — sleek, powerful, responsive. Now imagine driving it off the lot without ever reading the owner's manual. Sure, you can figure out how to steer and accelerate, but without understanding the maintenance schedule, the right fuel, or how to use the built-in systems, the car won't last. You'd burn out the engine, wear down the tires, and spend most of your time at the mechanic.

That's how most of us treat our bodies. We "drive" them from childhood through adulthood without ever really learning the basics of operation, maintenance, or troubleshooting. We assume that because our body keeps going, it must be fine — until one day the "check engine" light flashes as pain, fatigue, or illness.

A **manual** gives you three things:

1. **Orientation** — what this machine is, what it can do, and where its main systems are.
2. **Operation** — how to run it properly, from fueling (nutrition) to performance (exercise) to rest (recovery).
3. **Maintenance** — how to spot early signs of wear and tear, and how to prevent small problems from becoming major breakdowns.

Think of this book as the **owner's manual for your body** — written in plain language, with fewer technical diagrams and more practical instructions.

How to Use This Manual for Maximum Benefit

The purpose of this book isn't to overwhelm you with dense medical jargon or bury you in textbook-style details. It's to give you **usable knowledge** — the kind you can apply tomorrow, in the gym, at the dinner table, or even at your desk during a stressful workday.

Here's how to approach it:

1. Think Systems, Not Parts

Your body isn't just a pile of disconnected pieces. Bones, muscles, nerves, and hormones all work as **interdependent systems**. When one system thrives, others benefit; when one struggles, the rest compensate (sometimes poorly).

Instead of memorizing isolated facts ("the quadriceps extend the knee"), focus on how systems cooperate ("strong quadriceps reduce stress on the knee joint"). This perspective makes learning intuitive.

2. Learn Just Enough Science to Be Dangerous (in a Good Way)

You don't need a PhD in physiology to care for your body. But you do need a working understanding of the basics — how nutrition fuels energy, how muscles adapt to stress, how sleep resets your brain. Each chapter will give you the **essential principles** with clear analogies, so you can make informed choices without needing to Google every decision.

3. Apply, Don't Just Read

This isn't meant to be a book you read once and shelve. Each section comes with **practical takeaways** — daily habits, quick checklists, or troubleshooting guides you can apply right away. Think of it like the "Quick Start Guide" tucked inside a gadget box: you can skim and act today.

4. Check the Troubleshooting Section

Later chapters will serve as your "repair guide" — covering common issues like fatigue, injuries, and warning signs. Flip there anytime something feels off, the same way you'd look up a dashboard light in your car manual.

5. Respect the Warranty (Longevity Matters)

You may not be able to trade in your body, but you *can* extend its warranty. Think of your lifestyle choices as the difference between a car that runs smoothly for 300,000 miles and one that falls apart after 60,000. How you fuel, move, and maintain your body determines its lifespan and performance.

The Big Picture: From Basic Operation to Peak Performance

This manual is structured to mimic how you'd learn about any advanced machine:

- **Chapter 1–3: Orientation**
- **Chapters 4–9: Core Systems & How They Work**
- **Chapters 10–13: Maintenance & Upgrades**
- **Chapters 14–17: Troubleshooting & Repairs**
- **Chapters 18–20: Optimization & Longevity**
- **Chapters 21–22: Beyond Standard Use**

By the end, you'll understand not only *what's under the hood*, but also **how to keep it running at its best for decades to come**.

The Mindset Shift: From Passenger to Pilot

Most people live like **passengers** inside their own body. They go wherever it takes them, reacting when problems arise but rarely steering the course. This manual is about shifting you into the **pilot's seat**.

When you understand your body's systems, you can:

- Recognize when fatigue is simply a need for better fuel versus an early sign of burnout.
- Train smarter, not just harder, by respecting biomechanics.
- Make nutrition decisions that fuel performance rather than sabotage it.
- Catch minor issues before they spiral into chronic problems.
- Appreciate your body not as a burden to drag through life, but as a partner in everything you want to accomplish.

You didn't get to choose this machine. You didn't get to customize its specs or select optional features. And yet, you're the sole owner, operator, and caretaker of the most advanced piece of engineering ever created.

No matter where you're starting from — young or old, fit or struggling, confident or curious — you can **learn to run your body better**. This manual won't make you a doctor or an engineer, but it will give you something even more powerful: the ability to **understand and influence your own performance, health, and longevity**.

So, buckle up. Your orientation is complete. In the next chapters, we'll pop the hood and start exploring the systems that make you, **you**.

Chapter 2

Specifications & Design Overview

Every advanced machine begins with a spec sheet. Before you operate a high-performance car, computer, or aircraft, you want to know its core stats: size, weight, range, power output, fuel efficiency, and operating limits. Your body is no different.

Of course, humans aren't stamped out of a factory assembly line. Your "machine" comes with custom settings, influenced by genetics, environment, lifestyle, and time. Still, across the species, we share a remarkably consistent set of **baseline specifications** — universal features that make the human body the astonishing system it is.

In this chapter, we'll break down the core numbers, then zoom in on what makes this "hardware" and "software" blend unique: the seamless integration of **anatomy** (structure), **physiology** (function), and **biomechanics** (movement).

Key Stats: Size, Weight, and Performance Ranges

Let's start with some numbers — the vital statistics of your human body.

General Dimensions

- **Height range:** Average adult humans measure between **5'0" and 6'2" (152–188 cm)**, though the recorded range extends from under 2 feet (primordial dwarfism) to over 8 feet (gigantism).
- **Weight range:** A "healthy" average adult body weight varies widely, from **100 to 250 pounds (45–113 kg)** depending on sex, bone density, muscle mass, and fat distribution.

- **Surface area:** Spread flat, the skin of an average adult covers about **1.5–2 square meters** (roughly the size of a large bedsheet).

Power & Energy

- **Resting power output:** The body at rest burns about **80–100 watts** of energy — the equivalent of a dim light bulb.
- **Peak power output:** In short bursts, elite athletes can generate over **2,000 watts**, about the same as a professional cyclist during a sprint.
- **Daily fuel requirement:** Depending on activity, the average adult needs **1,600–3,000 kilocalories** per day — roughly the equivalent of burning through a liter of premium fuel.

Circulation & Respiratory Specs

- **Heart rate:** Ranges from **60–100 beats per minute** at rest, with elite endurance athletes dipping as low as **30–40 bpm**.
- **Cardiac output:** At peak exertion, the heart can pump over **20 liters of blood per minute** — enough to fill a large soda bottle every three seconds.
- **Breathing rate:** About **12–20 breaths per minute at rest**, scaling up to **40–60 breaths per minute during maximal exertion**.

Materials & Construction

- **Bone:** Ounce for ounce, stronger than concrete, yet lightweight and self-repairing.
- **Muscle:** Makes up **30–40% of body weight**, providing both motion and metabolic stability.
- **Skin:** The largest organ, weighing about **6 pounds (2.7 kg)**, renewing itself every **28–40 days**.
- **Water content:** Approximately **60% of total body weight** — meaning an average 150 lb adult carries about 90 lbs of water.

Spec Sheet Snapshot

System	Performance Range	Notes
Brain	20 watts of power use, 86 billion neurons	Faster than any supercomputer in parallel processing
Heart	100,000 beats/day; 2.5 billion beats in a lifetime	Pumps 1.5 gallons/min at rest, 5+ gallons/min at exercise
Lungs	6 liters of capacity; 500 million alveoli	Surface area equal to a tennis court
Muscles	600+ muscles; 30–40% of body weight	Adaptable, self-repairing
Bones	206 in adults, self-healing, dynamic remodeling	Stronger than steel by weight

System	Performance Range	Notes
Skin	1.5–2 m² surface area; first line of defense	Regenerates monthly
Fuel Efficiency	1,600–3,000 kcal/day (average adult)	Equivalent to ~1 liter of gasoline energy

The Unique Blend of Anatomy, Physiology, and Biomechanics

A car has an engine, a frame, and a transmission. A computer has hardware, software, and peripherals. The human body's design integrates **three interlocking layers of engineering**:

1. **Anatomy (the blueprint)** – What the parts are and how they're arranged.
2. **Physiology (the operations manual)** – What the parts do, and how they function in real time.
3. **Biomechanics (the movement physics)** – How forces, levers, and motion interact to create performance.

Each layer is impressive alone. But the true marvel lies in **integration** — anatomy creates the architecture, physiology powers it, and biomechanics turns it into coordinated movement.

1. Anatomy – The Blueprint

Anatomy is the **schematic drawing** of the human body. It's the "parts list" and "assembly diagram" that shows where bones, muscles, nerves, and organs sit.

Key elements of this blueprint:

- **Skeletal frame:** 206 bones provide structure, protection, and leverage.
- **Muscular layers:** 600+ muscles arranged for both power (quadriceps, glutes) and precision (small hand muscles, eye muscles).
- **Circulatory and respiratory systems:** Pipes, pumps, and filters distributing life-sustaining oxygen and nutrients.
- **Nervous system wiring:** An intricate web stretching across every square inch of the body.
- **Protective casing:** Skin, fascia, and connective tissue forming the outer shell.

The blueprint itself is **astonishingly efficient**: bones are hollow to maximize strength-to-weight ratio, muscles overlap for redundancy, and nerves branch like tree roots to ensure communication reaches every cell.

---

2. Physiology – The Operations Manual

Anatomy tells you where the parts are. **Physiology tells you what they do.**

Think of physiology as the **real-time operating system** of the human body.

- **The heart doesn't just sit there — it dynamically adjusts output** based on activity, stress, or rest.
- **The lungs aren't passive balloons — they actively regulate gas exchange** depending on oxygen demand.
- **Muscles don't just contract — they remodel themselves** in response to load, adapting to grow stronger, more efficient, or more enduring.
- **The endocrine system doesn't just release hormones — it fine-tunes balance across metabolism, growth, mood, and reproduction.**

Every organ is part of a **feedback loop**, constantly listening, responding, and adapting. Unlike most machines, which require manual tuning, the body **auto-adjusts** hundreds of variables every second without conscious input.

---

3. Biomechanics – The Physics of Movement

If anatomy is the parts list and physiology is the operations, then **biomechanics is the motion physics**.

Biomechanics is the study of **how forces interact with your body**: how joints act as levers, muscles generate torque, and tissues absorb shock.

- **Levers and pulleys:** Your bones act as rigid levers, while muscles and tendons act like ropes and pulleys.
- **Energy transfer:** Every stride, jump, or swing uses stored elastic energy in tendons and fascia — nature's springs.
- **Balance and stability:** Your nervous system integrates sensory input (from the inner ear, eyes, and proprioceptors) to keep you upright.
- **Efficiency:** A cheetah may run faster, but humans are built for **endurance efficiency**. Our upright gait and sweat-cooling system allow us to run marathons in heat where most animals would collapse.

Biomechanics also explains why **form matters**. A squat isn't just bending your knees — it's a precise orchestration of hip hinge, knee tracking, ankle mobility, and spinal stabilization. Done well, it's safe and powerful. Done poorly, it stresses joints and tissues.

Integration: More Than the Sum of Its Parts

The brilliance of the human body is not anatomy, physiology, or biomechanics alone, but the way they blend.

Consider running:

- Anatomy provides bones, muscles, tendons, and lungs.
- Physiology fuels them with oxygen, manages energy, and keeps internal balance.
- Biomechanics organizes movement into an efficient stride that conserves energy and minimizes wear.

You don't have to think about it consciously — the integration happens automatically. Yet, by **understanding each layer**, you can influence performance, prevent breakdowns, and fine-tune efficiency.

Why These Specs Matter

Why should you care about stats like heart rate ranges, oxygen uptake, or lever systems? Because **they define your limits and your potential**.

- Know your **engine capacity** (cardiovascular endurance), and you'll know how far you can push before burnout.
- Understand your **frame specs** (bone density, joint stability), and you'll prevent injury by training smarter.
- Learn the **fuel mix requirements** (nutrition and hydration), and you'll boost performance instead of sabotaging it.

- Recognize the **maintenance schedule** (recovery, sleep, check-ups), and you'll extend the warranty on your body far beyond the average.

This chapter's takeaway is simple: **Your body has specs. Learn them, respect them, and you'll unlock both performance and longevity.**

Every machine comes with limitations — speed governors, temperature ranges, wear tolerances. But the human body is unique because its **specs are adaptable**. With training, rest, and nutrition, you can **upgrade** your output, strengthen your frame, and extend your range.

You're not just operating the machine — you're also the engineer, mechanic, and driver. And with this manual in hand, you'll be equipped to treat the body not as a black box, but as the masterpiece of design it truly is.

Chapter 3

Safety Warnings & Operating Limits

Every advanced machine ships with a set of warnings: *"Do not operate above this temperature." "Keep away from water." "Replace worn parts on schedule."* These cautions aren't there to limit your fun — they're there to keep the machine running safely and effectively.

Your human body is no different. While it's the most adaptable, durable, and resilient piece of engineering you'll ever own, it still has **operating limits**. Push those limits without respect, and you risk breakdowns — sometimes minor and temporary, sometimes catastrophic and permanent.

In this chapter, we'll explore the essentials of **injury prevention** and the **environmental factors** that can push your body beyond its design envelope. Think of this as the red warning stickers in your owner's manual — the things to know before you rev the engine or take it into extreme conditions.

Injury Prevention Basics

The human body is self-repairing, but it's not indestructible. Most injuries happen when we ignore the body's warning signs or operate outside of its safe range.

1. Respect Load Limits

- **Bones and joints have thresholds.**
  Just like an aircraft wing can only flex so far before metal fatigue sets in, your joints and bones have limits. Too much load too quickly — think lifting a weight far beyond your training — can lead to sprains, fractures, or dislocations.
- **Progressive overload is key.**
  The body *can* grow stronger, but only if stress is increased gradually. Adding 5–10% more

resistance or distance per week is safe. Doubling overnight is not.

---

2. Warm-Up = Pre-Flight Check

You wouldn't launch a rocket cold. You shouldn't launch into exercise cold either.

- **Dynamic warm-ups** (leg swings, arm circles, light jogging) prepare muscles and joints by increasing blood flow.
- **Neurological priming** wakes up your nervous system so movements are coordinated and responsive.
- **Temperature boost:** A warmed-up muscle is more elastic, less likely to tear.

Skipping this step is like taking off in an icy plane — your system isn't ready for performance.

---

3. Mind the Form, Not Just the Effort

Bad form is like misaligning gears in a transmission: it works for a while, then grinds down components.

- **Posture matters:** Neutral spine, joint alignment, and controlled range of motion reduce stress.
- **Compensation warning:** If one muscle is weak or tight, others compensate, creating

imbalances. Over time, this leads to breakdowns (knee pain from weak hips, back pain from poor core stability).
- **Slow down:** Perfecting form at moderate intensity is more valuable than rushing into high intensity with sloppy technique.

---

4. The Importance of Recovery

Every mechanical system needs downtime. Airplanes undergo scheduled inspections; cars require oil changes. Your body requires **rest and repair**.

- **Microdamage heals stronger.** Muscles adapt by repairing tiny tears. Without rest, those microtears accumulate into injury.
- **Sleep is non-negotiable.** Growth hormone release, tissue repair, and nervous system recalibration all occur during deep sleep.
- **Active recovery:** Walking, stretching, and light movement boost circulation without adding more stress.

Ignoring recovery is like driving nonstop without ever pulling into a service station — eventually, the engine seizes.

5. Listen to the Dashboard Lights

Your body sends warning signals, much like indicator lights on a car:

- **Pain = check engine light.** Pain is not "weakness leaving the body." It's feedback. Persistent pain means something is wrong.
- **Swelling or stiffness = overheating light.** Inflammation is the body's cooling system; it's fine short-term, but if chronic, it signals overload.
- **Fatigue = low fuel light.** Persistent exhaustion means your system is running beyond its sustainable range.

Smart operators don't ignore warning lights. Neither should you.

Environmental Factors

Beyond injury from movement itself, the **environment** you operate in places unique demands on your machine. Extreme temperature, altitude, and hydration status all affect performance — sometimes drastically.

1. Temperature

Humans are warm-blooded machines with a narrow operating range. The body works best at a **core temperature of ~98.6°F (37°C)**.

Heat Stress

- **Sweat cooling:** The body regulates temperature by sweating. Each bead of sweat carries heat away as it evaporates.
- **Danger zone:** High humidity prevents evaporation, leading to overheating.
- **Heat exhaustion vs. heat stroke:**
    - *Heat exhaustion* = dizziness, rapid heartbeat, heavy sweating.
    - *Heat stroke* = core temperature >104°F, confusion, risk of organ failure. This is a medical emergency.

Cold Stress

- **Shivering:** Muscles contract rapidly to generate heat.
- **Vasoconstriction:** Blood flow pulls inward to preserve core organs. Extremities get cold first.
- **Hypothermia:** Prolonged exposure drops core temp below 95°F, leading to impaired coordination, slowed cognition, and eventually unconsciousness.

Practical Safety Notes

- Dress in layers in cold, light and breathable in heat.
- Acclimate gradually; don't go from air conditioning to running a marathon in 95°F weather.
- Stay hydrated — your cooling system depends on it.

---

2. Altitude

At sea level, the air is dense with oxygen molecules. As you climb higher, the air thins, reducing available oxygen.

- **Above 5,000 ft (1,500 m):** Some notice shortness of breath.
- **Above 8,000 ft (2,400 m):** Performance begins to decline noticeably.
- **Above 12,000 ft (3,600 m):** Acute Mountain Sickness risk increases — headaches, nausea, dizziness.
- **Extreme altitudes (18,000+ ft / 5,500+ m):** Supplemental oxygen becomes necessary for most people.

The body does adapt — by producing more red blood cells to carry oxygen — but acclimatization takes **days to weeks**. Without it, risk of altitude sickness or pulmonary/cerebral edema rises.

3. Hydration

Water is the body's most critical fluid. At ~60% of body weight, it lubricates joints, regulates temperature, aids digestion, and powers cellular processes.

- **Mild dehydration (1–2% body weight lost):** Thirst, reduced performance, impaired focus.
- **Moderate dehydration (3–5%):** Fatigue, headache, elevated heart rate, risk of heat illness.
- **Severe dehydration (6–10%+):** Confusion, collapse, kidney stress, life-threatening.

Key facts:

- The average adult loses **2–3 liters of water/day** through sweat, urine, and breathing — more in heat or exercise.
- Thirst lags behind dehydration, so **waiting to feel thirsty is too late**.
- Electrolytes (sodium, potassium, magnesium) are essential for fluid balance. Sweat isn't just water — it's a salt solution.

Practical Safety Notes

- Drink consistently throughout the day, not just at meals.
- For exercise longer than 60 minutes, supplement water with electrolytes.
- Monitor urine color — pale yellow = hydrated, dark amber = low fuel warning.

Safe Operating Limits

Every system has boundaries. Push too far, and efficiency turns into danger.

- **Temperature:** Core body temp should stay between **95–104°F (35–40°C)**. Outside of this, performance fails and risk skyrockets.
- **Hydration:** Keep fluid balance within **1–2% of body weight loss**. Beyond that, endurance and cognition deteriorate.
- **Oxygen availability:** Your body thrives at sea level but requires adaptation above **8,000 ft**.
- **Load:** Muscles and bones can adapt to extraordinary strength, but only with **progressive training**. Sudden extremes invite injury.

Think of these as your **operating envelope**. The human body is highly adaptable, but not limitless. Respect the ranges, and the system thrives. Ignore them, and you risk catastrophic failure.

Safety warnings may sound restrictive, but they're really about freedom. The more you understand your limits, the more confidently you can push them — climbing higher, running farther, training harder, exploring hotter or colder environments — without fear of breakdown.

Injury prevention and environmental awareness aren't about holding back. They're about **unlocking sustainable performance**. When you learn how to operate within safe ranges, you gain the confidence to test your edges, explore new environments, and get the most out of the world's most advanced piece of engineering: your human body.

Part 2

Core Systems

&

How They Work

Chapter 4

The Frame: Skeletal System

The Engineering of Your Frame

Every machine has a frame — a chassis, skeleton, or supporting structure that gives it shape and allows other components to function. Cars have steel frames, airplanes have fuselages, and skyscrapers have steel and concrete cores.

For the human body, the frame is the **skeletal system**. It's not just scaffolding to hang muscles on — it's a **living, dynamic, constantly adapting tissue**. Unlike a car frame, which rusts and weakens over time, your bones are **self-repairing, self-remodeling, and capable of strengthening under stress**.

This chapter explores how the skeletal system is built, how its joints create movement, and how you can maintain bone health for a lifetime of strong, reliable performance.

Structure of the Skeletal System

1. The Blueprint

- **Number of bones:** The adult skeleton consists of **206 bones**, though infants are born with ~270. As you grow, many fuse (like the skull and pelvis).
- **Categories:**
    - *Axial skeleton* (80 bones): skull, spine, rib cage — the protective core.
    - *Appendicular skeleton* (126 bones): arms, legs, pelvis, shoulders — the levers of movement.
- **Composition:** Bone is a composite material of **collagen (for flexibility)** and **hydroxyapatite mineral crystals (for hardness)**, giving it the strength of reinforced concrete but with resilience.

2. The Spine – Central Support Column

The spine is your body's **master beam**:

- **33 vertebrae in total:** 7 cervical, 12 thoracic, 5 lumbar, 5 sacral (fused), 4 coccygeal (tailbone).
- **Shock absorption:** Intervertebral discs act as cushions and spacers, allowing flexibility while absorbing impact.
- **Curves as engineering design:** The natural S-curve distributes weight evenly and reduces stress, just like arches in bridges.

---

3. The Rib Cage & Skull – Protective Housing

- **Rib cage:** 24 ribs plus sternum, forming a protective cage for lungs and heart. The ribs expand and contract with breathing — a moving shield.
- **Skull:** 22 bones fused into a rigid helmet, protecting the brain. Jaws and facial bones allow eating, breathing, and expression.

---

4. The Limbs – Levers of Motion

Arms and legs are **lever systems** designed for movement:

- **Upper limb:** Shoulder girdle, humerus, radius, ulna, and hand bones allow reach and fine motor control.
- **Lower limb:** Pelvis, femur, tibia, fibula, and foot bones create stability and locomotion.
- **Feet:** 26 bones per foot, with arches that act like suspension bridges, storing and releasing energy with each step.

Joints: Movement at the Connections

Bones alone are rigid. **Joints** give the skeleton mobility. Think of them as **hinges, ball-and-socket mounts, and swivels** in a complex machine.

Types of Joints

- **Fixed joints:** Like the fused plates of the skull — designed for protection, not movement.
- **Cartilaginous joints:** Allow limited movement (e.g., between vertebrae).
- **Synovial joints:** Highly mobile, fluid-filled, and most important for movement.

Synovial Joint Subtypes

- **Hinge joint:** Elbows, knees — movement in one plane.

- **Ball-and-socket joint:** Shoulder, hip — wide range of motion.
- **Pivot joint:** Neck (turning head side to side).
- **Gliding joint:** Wrists and ankles.
- **Saddle joint:** Thumb — unique mobility enabling gripping.

Load-Bearing Capacity

- **Bones are weight-class champions.**
    - Femur (thigh bone) can withstand compressive forces up to **1,800–2,500 lbs** before breaking.
    - Spine discs can tolerate hundreds of pounds of compression but weaken under poor posture or sudden overload.
- **Distribution matters.** Proper alignment spreads force across multiple bones and joints. Misalignment (e.g., bad squat form) can overload one structure, leading to injury.

Bone Health & Maintenance

Your skeleton isn't static — it's in constant motion at the microscopic level. Every day, bone tissue is broken down by cells called **osteoclasts** and rebuilt by **osteoblasts**. This process, called **remodeling**, ensures that bones adapt to stress and stay strong.

1. Stress & Adaptation

- **Wolff's Law:** Bones adapt to the loads placed on them. Stress them with weight-bearing exercise, and they grow denser. Remove stress (bed rest, sedentary living), and they weaken.
- **Examples:**
    - Tennis players often have a thicker, denser serving arm bone.
    - Astronauts lose bone density in microgravity without exercise countermeasures.

---

2. Nutrition for Bones

- **Calcium:** The primary building block of bone mineral. Found in dairy, leafy greens, fortified foods.
- **Vitamin D:** Essential for calcium absorption. Sunlight and supplementation often required.
- **Protein:** Provides collagen framework for bone strength.
- **Other minerals:** Magnesium, phosphorus, and zinc all support bone integrity.

---

3. Hormonal Influence

- **Estrogen and testosterone:** Critical for bone density. Low hormone levels (e.g., post-menopause) increase osteoporosis risk.

- **Parathyroid hormone & calcitonin:** Regulate calcium levels, maintaining balance between bone breakdown and formation.

---

4. Lifestyle Factors

- **Exercise:** Weight-bearing activities (walking, running, lifting, jumping) stimulate bone growth. Swimming and cycling improve fitness but don't build bone density as effectively.
- **Posture & alignment:** Proper movement mechanics reduce uneven wear.
- **Sleep:** Growth hormone release during deep sleep aids bone remodeling.
- **Avoiding negatives:** Smoking, excessive alcohol, and chronic stress hormones (cortisol) weaken bones.

---

5. Age & Bone Health

- **Peak bone mass:** Reached in late 20s. After that, maintenance is key.
- **Decline with age:** Bones lose density naturally, but strength training, proper nutrition, and lifestyle habits slow this decline.
- **Osteoporosis:** A disease of fragile, porous bones — preventable through proactive care decades earlier.

Operating Tips for the Skeletal Frame

Think of this as your **"maintenance checklist"** for the skeleton:

1. **Daily load-bearing activity:** Walk, lift, climb stairs. Use your bones or lose them.
2. **Fuel properly:** Get adequate calcium, vitamin D, and protein.
3. **Avoid overload:** Respect alignment, posture, and form.
4. **Check wear & tear:** Persistent joint pain, fractures, or posture changes are early warning lights.
5. **Regular service checks:** Bone density scans (DEXA) recommended for those at risk (especially women post-menopause).

Your skeleton isn't just scaffolding — it's a **living, evolving engineering marvel**. Strong bones and healthy joints are the foundation of every athletic movement, every daily task, and every adventure you'll ever undertake.

Respect the structure, maintain it wisely, and your frame will support you with strength and resilience for decades. Neglect it, and even the most powerful muscles or sharpest mind will be limited by a weakened chassis.

The good news? Unlike machines made of steel or aluminum, your frame **adapts**. With proper stress, fuel, and care, you can make your skeleton stronger year after year — ensuring that the world's most advanced engineering continues to hold you up, protect you, and move you forward.

Chapter 5

The Engine: Muscular System

The Power Plant of Your Machine

Every machine needs an engine — a system to convert fuel into motion. In cars, it's the combustion engine; in computers, it's the processor; in rockets, it's the propulsion system.

For the human body, the **muscular system** is the engine. More than 600 muscles work together to generate power, stabilize joints, move blood, support posture, and even regulate body temperature. Muscles are not just bundles of tissue — they are **living engines**: self-repairing, adaptable, and capable of producing astonishing amounts of force relative to their size.

This chapter explores how your muscular system is structured, how it produces movement, the different types of muscles, and how you can maintain this engine for peak performance and longevity.

Structure of the Muscular System

1. Composition and Organization

Muscles are built from layers of structure:

- **Muscle fibers:** Long, threadlike cells capable of contraction.
- **Myofibrils:** Bundles inside each fiber, containing actin and myosin — the sliding filaments that generate force.
- **Fascicles:** Groups of fibers bundled together by connective tissue.
- **Whole muscle:** Hundreds or thousands of fascicles working as a single unit.

This layered arrangement allows muscles to be **incredibly strong yet finely controlled**. Your quadriceps can squat hundreds of pounds, while tiny eye muscles can move with millimeter precision.

---

2. Types of Muscle Tissue

The body has **three major types of muscle**, each with a unique role:

- **Skeletal muscle:** Voluntary, striated, attached to bones. These are the muscles you train in the gym — responsible for posture, locomotion, and force.
- **Cardiac muscle:** Found only in the heart. Involuntary, rhythmic, resistant to fatigue. It contracts about 100,000 times a day for your entire life.
- **Smooth muscle:** Involuntary, found in organs and blood vessels. It moves food through your intestines, regulates blood pressure, and controls pupil dilation.

For the purposes of this "user manual," our main focus is **skeletal muscle** — the engine you directly control.

Muscle Function and Performance

1. Contraction: How the Engine Fires

Muscle fibers contract through the **sliding filament mechanism**:

- Nerve signals release calcium inside the muscle.
- Myosin heads attach to actin filaments and pull them inward.
- This microscopic sliding shortens the muscle fiber, producing force.

Multiply this by billions of fibers working together, and you get movement ranging from a gentle handshake to a powerful deadlift.

---

2. Force and Endurance

Muscle performance depends on **fiber type distribution**:

- **Type I (slow-twitch):** Endurance specialists. Use oxygen efficiently, resist fatigue, ideal for distance running and posture.
- **Type IIa (fast-twitch oxidative):** Versatile. Moderate power and endurance.

- **Type IIb/x (fast-twitch glycolytic):** Pure power. Explosive, high-force, fatigue quickly. Perfect for sprinting and weightlifting.

Each person's mix is genetically determined, but training can shift performance. Marathon training builds endurance capacity; sprinting and lifting enhance fast-twitch power.

---

3. Muscles as Stabilizers

Not all muscles are about movement. Many function as **stabilizers**, keeping joints aligned and posture upright.

- The **core muscles** (abdominals, obliques, spinal stabilizers) protect the spine and allow efficient force transfer.
- **Hip stabilizers** keep knees tracking properly during running or squatting.
- **Rotator cuff muscles** secure the shoulder joint, preventing dislocation.

Think of stabilizers as the **mounts and brackets** holding your engine in place so it doesn't rattle itself apart.

Joints, Muscles, and Levers

Muscles and bones form a **lever system**.

- **Origin:** Where a muscle attaches to a stable bone.
- **Insertion:** Where it attaches to the bone it moves.
- **Action:** The movement produced when the muscle contracts.

Examples:

- The **biceps brachii** originates on the shoulder and inserts on the forearm. Contraction flexes the elbow.
- The **quadriceps** straighten the knee by pulling on the tibia through the patellar tendon.

This lever system allows enormous versatility: fine movements like typing, powerful actions like jumping, and endurance feats like marathon running.

Load-Bearing Capacity

Muscles are **power-to-weight champions**:

- **Relative strength:** A 150 lb gymnast can hold their body weight upside down on one arm.

- **Absolute strength:** A few elite powerlifters have squat over 1,000 lbs.
- **Efficiency:** At rest, muscles consume little energy. When activated, they can increase metabolism 10- to 20-fold.

But every engine has limits:

- **Overtraining** leads to fatigue, breakdown, and even rhabdomyolysis (serious muscle tissue damage).
- **Poor mechanics** overload joints and connective tissue, leading to injury.

Muscle Health & Maintenance

1. Training Principles

- **Progressive overload:** Gradually increase resistance or intensity to stimulate adaptation.
- **Specificity:** Train the qualities you want (endurance vs. strength vs. power).
- **Variation:** Mix intensity, volume, and exercise selection to prevent stagnation.
- **Recovery:** Muscles adapt during rest, not during the workout itself.

2. Fuel for the Engine

Muscles are fuel-flexible, but proper nutrition optimizes performance:

- **Carbohydrates:** Primary quick-burning fuel for high-intensity work. Stored as glycogen in muscles and liver.
- **Fats:** Slow-burning fuel for endurance. Each pound of body fat stores ~3,500 kcal.
- **Protein:** Builds and repairs muscle tissue. Not ideal as a primary fuel but essential for maintenance.
- **Micronutrients:** Magnesium, potassium, calcium support contraction and recovery.

---

3. Rest and Recovery

- **Microtears repair stronger:** Training creates small tears in muscle fibers. Recovery rebuilds them thicker and stronger.
- **Sleep:** Deep sleep is when growth hormone and testosterone peak, driving repair.
- **Active recovery:** Low-intensity movement increases circulation, flushing out byproducts.

---

4. Age and Muscle Maintenance

- **Sarcopenia:** Age-related muscle loss begins around age 30, accelerating after 50.

- **Countermeasures:** Resistance training and high-protein diets dramatically slow this decline.
- **Function over bulk:** Even modest strength gains preserve independence and reduce fall risk in aging adults.

Common Muscle Issues

- **Cramps:** Sudden involuntary contractions, often due to dehydration, fatigue, or electrolyte imbalance.
- **Strains:** Overstretching or tearing fibers.
- **Delayed Onset Muscle Soreness (DOMS):** Microdamage after unaccustomed exercise. Normal, but should subside in 24–72 hours.
- **Imbalances:** Overdeveloping one muscle group (e.g., chest vs. back) creates postural issues. Balance training matters.

Operating Tips for Your Muscular Engine

Think of these as your **muscle maintenance checklist**:

1. **Move daily:** Use muscles through their full range. Inactivity = engine rust.
2. **Train strength 2–3x/week:** Preserve muscle and bone density.
3. **Fuel wisely:** Adequate protein, hydration, and balanced macros.
4. **Respect form:** Quality of movement beats ego lifting.
5. **Prioritize recovery:** Sleep and rest are mandatory, not optional.
6. **Balance the system:** Train push/pull, flexion/extension, left/right sides equally.

Your muscles are not just the body's engine — they're also its **shock absorbers, posture supports, and metabolic regulators**. They are living engines, capable of adapting to whatever demands you place on them.

Train them, fuel them, and give them time to recover, and they'll deliver performance far beyond what you might imagine. Neglect them, and the world's most advanced frame loses its power source.

Chapter 6

The Wiring: Nervous System

The Control Center

Every high-performance machine has wiring and circuitry. A car's engine control unit coordinates spark plugs, sensors, and fuel injectors. A computer's processor sends signals through circuits to run programs.

For the human body, the **nervous system** is both **the wiring** (nerves that transmit signals) and **the operating software** (the brain and spinal cord that process and direct those signals). Without it, your muscular engine never fires, your skeletal frame sits idle, and your organs lose coordination.

This chapter will explore the structure of the nervous system, how signals travel, how it integrates with muscles and senses, and how to maintain its health for performance and longevity.

Structure of the Nervous System

1. Central Nervous System (CNS)

- **Brain:** The ultimate control tower. Weighs ~3 pounds, runs on ~20 watts of power, yet outperforms any supercomputer in parallel processing.
- **Spinal cord:** The main trunk line, ~18 inches long, protected by vertebrae. It carries signals to and from the brain and manages reflexes.

2. Peripheral Nervous System (PNS)

- **Sensory nerves (afferent):** Carry input from sensors (eyes, ears, skin, joints).
- **Motor nerves (efferent):** Deliver output from the brain/spinal cord to muscles and glands.

- **Autonomic division:** Regulates involuntary functions — heart rate, digestion, temperature. Subdivided into:
  - *Sympathetic system:* "Fight or flight." Speeds heart, increases alertness.
  - *Parasympathetic system:* "Rest and digest." Calms the body, aids recovery.

3. Neurons – The Wiring Units

- **86 billion neurons in the brain alone.**
- Each neuron communicates via **electrical impulses** (action potentials) and **chemical messengers** (neurotransmitters).
- Connection points (synapses) form vast circuits — estimated at 100 trillion in number.

How Signals Travel

Imagine electrical wiring in a house. The nervous system uses a similar principle, but with more complexity:

- **Resting potential:** A neuron maintains a negative charge inside compared to outside.
- **Action potential:** A rapid "flip" of charge propagates down the axon like a spark along a wire.
- **Myelin insulation:** Fatty sheaths around axons speed signal conduction, similar to insulation on copper wire.

- **Synapses:** At the end, neurotransmitters bridge the gap to the next neuron or muscle cell, transmitting the signal.

Speed ranges from **1 mph (in unmyelinated fibers)** to over **250 mph (in fast motor fibers)**. This allows you to pull your hand from a hot stove in milliseconds or track a flying ball in real time.

Integration with the Body

1. Motor Control

- Signals from the motor cortex travel down the spinal cord to motor neurons.
- Motor units (a nerve + the muscle fibers it controls) determine precision.
    - Eye muscles: 1 neuron for ~10 fibers (high precision).
    - Leg muscles: 1 neuron for ~1,000 fibers (high power).

2. Sensory Feedback

- **Proprioceptors:** Sensors in muscles, tendons, and joints tell the brain where the body is in space.
- **Balance sensors:** Inner ear structures detect acceleration and orientation.
- **Touch, pain, temperature receptors:** Provide protective and environmental feedback.

3. Reflexes

- Some responses bypass the brain for speed. Example: the knee-jerk reflex occurs entirely at the spinal cord level. Reflexes act like **automatic circuit breakers** to prevent damage.

Performance Ranges

The nervous system defines your operating performance:

- **Reaction time:** Average = ~200 ms; elite athletes can react in ~120 ms.
- **Nerve conduction speed:** Up to 120 m/s in myelinated fibers.
- **Plasticity:** The brain can rewire itself after injury or training — unique among biological systems.

Just like updating a computer's operating system, the nervous system adapts with practice. Repetition of skills strengthens neural circuits ("neurons that fire together, wire together").

Maintenance & Health of the Nervous System

1. Fuel & Energy

- The brain consumes ~20% of daily calories. Glucose is its primary fuel, but ketones can substitute in fasting or low-carb states.
- Hydration is critical — even 2% dehydration reduces cognitive function.

2. Sleep & Recovery

- Sleep clears metabolic waste from the brain via the glymphatic system.
- Deep sleep consolidates memory and enhances motor learning.

3. Training the Nervous System

- **Strength training:** Improves neural recruitment of muscle fibers before muscle size increases.
- **Skill practice:** Refines coordination by optimizing neural pathways.
- **Balance & agility drills:** Enhance proprioception and reflex speed.

4. Protective Maintenance

- **Avoid chronic stress:** Prolonged sympathetic activation depletes reserves, increases blood pressure, weakens immunity.

- **Protect the head:** Helmets and safety matter; neurons do not regenerate easily.
- **Nutritional support:** Omega-3 fatty acids, B-vitamins, magnesium support nerve function.

Environmental Factors Affecting the Nervous System

- **Temperature extremes:** Heat can slow neural conduction; cold can numb and impair control.
- **Altitude:** Low oxygen impairs brain function, causing slowed reflexes, confusion, or poor coordination.
- **Toxins & substances:** Alcohol slows conduction, caffeine speeds alertness, some drugs interfere with neurotransmitters.

Common Issues & Troubleshooting

- **Nerve impingement:** Compression (e.g., herniated disc) causing pain, tingling, weakness.
- **Neuropathy:** Damage from diabetes, toxins, or injuries leading to numbness.

- **Multiple sclerosis:** Autoimmune attack on myelin insulation, slowing signals.
- **Burnout & fatigue:** Nervous system overload from chronic stress or overtraining.

Operating Tips for the Nervous System

1. **Prioritize sleep:** 7–9 hours nightly for cognitive and motor health.
2. **Fuel the brain:** Steady blood sugar, hydration, omega-3 fats.
3. **Challenge the wiring:** Learn new skills, puzzles, and movements to keep plasticity active.
4. **Balance load:** Alternate high stress ("fight or flight") with recovery ("rest and digest").
5. **Protect the circuits:** Safety gear, stress management, and ergonomic posture reduce wear.

Your nervous system is both the **wiring harness and the software** of your body. It integrates every system, allows split-second reactions, and stores the sum of your experiences and skills. Unlike mechanical wiring, it adapts and rewires itself continuously — a living system that grows stronger with use.

Respect your wiring, fuel it properly, and keep it challenged, and it will keep your muscular engine firing and your skeletal frame coordinated for a lifetime of performance.

Chapter 7

The Power Supply: Cardiovascular System

The Fuel Pump and Delivery Network

No machine runs without power. Cars need gasoline pumps, planes need fuel delivery lines, and computers need power supplies that distribute electricity across circuits.

In the human body, the **cardiovascular system** is the power supply and distribution network. It ensures that oxygen and nutrients reach every cell, while waste products like carbon dioxide are carried away. It is both **pump and plumbing**, running nonstop from your first heartbeat before birth until your last.

This chapter explores the structure of the cardiovascular system, its performance ranges, and how to maintain it for a lifetime of efficient fuel delivery.

The Structure of the Cardiovascular System

1. The Pump: The Heart

- **Size & weight:** About the size of your fist, weighing ~10–12 ounces.
- **Chambers:** Four rooms — two atria (receiving) and two ventricles (pumping).
- **Valves:** One-way doors (tricuspid, pulmonary, mitral, aortic) that ensure blood flows forward, never backward.
- **Fuel:** The heart muscle (myocardium) is unique — it contracts rhythmically and tirelessly, fed by its own coronary arteries.

The heart is the most reliable pump known: it contracts **~100,000 times a day**, moving about **2,000 gallons of blood daily**.

2. The Pipes: Blood Vessels

- **Arteries:** Thick-walled, high-pressure pipes carrying blood away from the heart.
- **Veins:** Thin-walled, low-pressure return lines with valves to prevent backflow.
- **Capillaries:** Microscopic exchange points — where oxygen and nutrients diffuse into tissues and waste products diffuse out.

Total length of this vascular plumbing? Roughly **60,000 miles** — enough to circle Earth twice.

---

3. The Fluid: Blood

- **Volume:** ~5 liters in an average adult.
- **Components:**
    - *Red blood cells:* Carry oxygen via hemoglobin.
    - *White blood cells:* Defend against infection.
    - *Platelets:* Aid clotting.
    - *Plasma:* The fluid matrix transporting nutrients, hormones, and waste.

Blood is not just fluid — it's a living, circulating tissue.

Performance Ranges

1. Heart Rate

- **Resting:** 60–100 beats per minute (bpm).
- **Athlete resting:** 30–50 bpm (due to efficiency).
- **Maximum:** Roughly 220 – age (formula-based). Elite athletes may sustain 190+ bpm under load.

2. Stroke Volume & Cardiac Output

- **Stroke volume:** Amount of blood pumped per beat (~70 mL at rest, up to 120 mL with training).
- **Cardiac output:** Stroke volume × heart rate. At rest ~5 L/min; during maximal exercise 20–40 L/min.

3. Blood Pressure

- **Normal:** ~120/80 mmHg.
- **High (hypertension):** Consistently >140/90 increases risk of stroke, heart attack.
- **Low:** <90/60 may cause dizziness, fainting.

How the System Works

1. Oxygen Delivery

- Blood picks up oxygen in the lungs.
- Hemoglobin in red blood cells binds oxygen molecules.
- Arteries deliver oxygen-rich blood to tissues.

2. Waste Removal

- Carbon dioxide diffuses back into the blood.
- Veins return it to the lungs for exhalation.
- Kidneys filter metabolic byproducts.

3. Circuits in Parallel

- **Systemic circulation:** Heart → body → heart.
- **Pulmonary circulation:** Heart → lungs → heart.
- Both loops run simultaneously, coordinated with every heartbeat.

Adaptability: Training the Pump

The cardiovascular system is not fixed — it adapts to training:

- **Endurance training:** Increases stroke volume, lowers resting heart rate, improves capillary density.
- **Strength training:** Raises blood pressure temporarily but enhances vascular resilience.
- **High-intensity intervals:** Boost VO_2 max — the maximum oxygen your body can use, a key fitness measure.

Athletes often show **athlete's heart**: larger chambers, stronger walls, and more efficient pumping.

Maintenance & Health of the Cardiovascular System

1. Nutrition

- **Healthy fats:** Omega-3s (fish, nuts) reduce inflammation and support vessel flexibility.
- **Limit trans fats & excess sodium:** Prevent clogged arteries and high blood pressure.
- **Antioxidants:** Fruits and vegetables protect vessels from oxidative stress.

2. Exercise

- Aerobic activity (walking, cycling, swimming) strengthens the heart muscle.
- Just **150 minutes/week of moderate exercise** reduces heart disease risk by up to 50%.

3. Recovery

- Stress management is vital: chronic stress keeps the sympathetic system active, straining the heart.
- Sleep supports blood pressure regulation and vascular repair.

Environmental Factors

1. Temperature

- **Heat:** Increases cardiovascular load as blood is diverted to skin for cooling.
- **Cold:** Constricts vessels, raising blood pressure.

2. Altitude

- Less oxygen available. The heart must pump harder. Over time, red blood cell count increases to compensate.

3. Hydration

- Blood volume depends on water. Dehydration lowers volume, stressing the heart.
- Even 2% dehydration reduces endurance performance.

Common Issues & Troubleshooting

- **Hypertension:** "Silent killer." Damages vessels, raises risk of stroke.
- **Atherosclerosis:** Plaque buildup narrowing arteries.
- **Arrhythmias:** Irregular rhythms, ranging from benign to life-threatening.
- **Heart failure:** Pumping capacity impaired.
- **Heart attack (myocardial infarction):** Blockage of coronary artery cutting off oxygen to heart muscle.

Operating Tips for the Cardiovascular System

1. **Move daily:** Even walking boosts circulation.
2. **Monitor numbers:** Check blood pressure, cholesterol, resting heart rate.
3. **Hydrate consistently:** Maintain blood volume.
4. **Fuel smart:** Favor whole foods, reduce processed excess.
5. **Manage stress:** Breathing, mindfulness, or downtime protect your heart.
6. **Don't smoke:** Smoking damages vessels and lowers oxygen delivery.

Your cardiovascular system is the **lifeblood of your machine** — literally. It fuels every cell, supports endurance, clears waste, and adapts to your activity level. Unlike a car's fuel pump, it cannot be swapped out when it fails. But the good news is, it's trainable. With proper fuel, consistent movement, and preventive care, your cardiovascular "power supply" can remain efficient for decades, giving you energy, stamina, and resilience.

Chapter 8

The Cooling & Waste Removal: Respiratory & Excretory Systems

The Body's AC, Exhaust, and Filter Systems

Every high-performance machine needs cooling and waste disposal. Engines overheat without radiators. Computers fry without fans. Cars stall without exhaust systems.

The human body is no different. To operate efficiently, it must:

1. **Cool itself** — regulate temperature so enzymes and cells work within a safe range.
2. **Bring in fresh fuel (oxygen)** and remove combustion byproducts (carbon dioxide).
3. **Filter out waste** like urea, salts, and toxins to keep the chemical environment stable.

This job falls to the **respiratory system** (the air intake, exhaust, and heat exchanger) and the **excretory system** (the filters and waste disposal units). Together, they keep the body balanced and safe under every condition from a casual stroll to a desert marathon.

The Respiratory System: Air Intake and Cooling

1. Structure

- **Airways:** Nose, mouth, pharynx, larynx, trachea — the intake pipes.
- **Bronchi and bronchioles:** Branching tubes leading into the lungs.
- **Alveoli:** Tiny sacs (~500 million of them) with a combined surface area the size of a tennis court, where oxygen enters blood and carbon dioxide exits.

2. Mechanics of Breathing

- **Inhalation:** Diaphragm contracts downward, ribs expand outward, drawing air in.
- **Exhalation:** Diaphragm relaxes, lungs recoil, pushing air out.
- **Ventilation rate:** ~12–20 breaths/minute at rest, up to 40–60/minute during maximal exertion.

3. Gas Exchange

- Oxygen diffuses into capillaries, binding to hemoglobin.
- Carbon dioxide diffuses from blood into alveoli, exhaled with the next breath.
- This constant exchange is as vital as fueling — without oxygen, the brain fails in 4–6 minutes.

Cooling Functions of the Respiratory System

Breathing isn't just about oxygen. It's part of the **cooling system**:

- **Evaporative cooling:** Exhaling moist air removes heat and water vapor.
- **Panting (in some animals):** Humans don't pant, but heavy breathing in heat still aids cooling.

- **Integration with sweat:** The respiratory system works with the skin's sweat glands to regulate body temperature.

During exercise, **20% of heat loss** can occur through respiration alone.

The Excretory System: Filters and Waste Disposal

1. Kidneys – The Primary Filters

- **Size:** About the size of fists, located near the lower back.
- **Function:** Filter ~50 gallons of blood daily, producing 1–2 quarts of urine.
- **Nephrons:** ~1 million per kidney. Each nephron filters blood, reabsorbs what's needed, and secretes waste.

2. Major Roles

- **Waste removal:** Urea (protein breakdown), uric acid, creatinine.
- **Fluid balance:** Adjust water levels to prevent dehydration or overhydration.
- **Electrolyte balance:** Maintain sodium, potassium, calcium, and magnesium levels for nerve and muscle function.

- **Blood pressure regulation:** Through hormones like renin.

3. Accessory Organs

- **Liver:** Detoxifies chemicals, processes nutrients, produces bile.
- **Skin:** Excretes water and salts through sweat.
- **Lungs:** Expel carbon dioxide (shared function).

Performance Ranges

Respiratory

- **Tidal volume (air per breath):** ~500 mL at rest; up to 3–4 liters at maximum effort.
- **Lung capacity:** ~6 liters total (varies by sex, size, and fitness).
- **Oxygen uptake (VO_2 max):** A critical measure of endurance. Elite athletes can hit 70–90 mL/kg/min; average adults ~30–40.

Excretory

- **Urine output:** 0.5–2 liters/day (hydration dependent).
- **Filtration rate:** Kidneys filter ~125 mL of blood per minute (glomerular filtration rate).
- **Sweat rate:** Can exceed 1–2 liters/hour in hot conditions or intense exercise.

Maintenance & Health

Respiratory Health

- **Avoid smoking/vaping:** These damage alveoli, reduce capacity, and increase cancer risk.
- **Train breathing:** Practices like diaphragmatic breathing, breath-hold drills, and endurance training improve lung efficiency.
- **Stay active:** Aerobic exercise increases capillary density and lung utilization.

Excretory Health

- **Hydration:** Adequate water intake keeps kidneys flushing waste efficiently.
- **Balanced diet:** Excessive processed sodium stresses kidneys and raises blood pressure.
- **Avoid toxins:** Overuse of NSAIDs, alcohol, or processed foods can overload the filtration system.
- **Monitor output:** Urine color is a simple diagnostic — pale yellow = hydrated; dark = dehydration.

Environmental Factors

Heat

- In hot environments, sweat output skyrockets, demanding more water and electrolytes.
- Risk: heat exhaustion, heat stroke, dehydration.

Cold

- Cold, dry air increases water loss through breathing.
- Kidneys may increase urine output ("cold diuresis"), which can worsen dehydration.

Altitude

- Thin air forces faster breathing. Increased ventilation dries out airways and accelerates water loss. Kidneys also adjust by excreting bicarbonate to help the blood adapt to reduced oxygen.

Common Issues & Troubleshooting

- **Asthma:** Narrowed airways cause wheezing and difficulty breathing.

- **Chronic obstructive pulmonary disease (COPD):** Long-term airway damage from smoking or pollutants.
- **Kidney stones:** Crystallized minerals blocking urine flow, causing severe pain.
- **Urinary tract infections:** Bacterial infection of bladder or urethra.
- **Dehydration:** Too little fluid intake or too much loss; can cause dizziness, cramps, and impaired cognition.

Operating Tips for the Cooling & Waste Systems

1. **Hydrate daily:** Don't wait for thirst.
2. **Monitor urine color:** A built-in indicator of hydration.
3. **Support your lungs:** Avoid smoking, keep airways clear, and train breathing efficiency.
4. **Manage environment:** Adjust clothing, pace, and fluid intake in heat/cold.
5. **Balance electrolytes:** Especially during extended exercise or heat exposure.
6. **Check warning lights:** Persistent shortness of breath, swelling, painful urination, or changes in urine output = service check needed.

Your respiratory and excretory systems are the **cooling fans and filters** of your body's design. They keep the internal environment stable, flush out waste, and protect you from overheating, dehydration, and toxic buildup. Like any advanced machine, these systems require **steady maintenance and awareness of operating limits**.

Respect them, and you'll maintain efficient cooling, clean fuel exchange, and smooth waste disposal for decades of performance. Ignore them, and the system clogs, overheats, or shuts down.

Chapter 9

The Control Panel: Endocrine & Immune Systems

Software Updates and Security Systems

Every advanced machine has two essential control features: **Software updates and regulators** that fine-tune performance and coordinate systems and **Firewalls and security**

systems that detect intruders and defend against threats.

In the human body, the **endocrine system** plays the role of software updater and regulator, releasing hormones that influence everything from growth and metabolism to stress and reproduction. The **immune system** serves as your internal security force, identifying harmful invaders (like viruses and bacteria), neutralizing them, and remembering threats for future defense.

Together, these two systems form the **control panel** — constantly monitoring, balancing, and adjusting to keep your machine in peak condition.

The Endocrine System: Software Updates

The endocrine system is made up of **glands that secrete hormones** — chemical messengers that travel through the bloodstream to regulate body functions. Unlike the rapid electrical signals of the nervous system, hormones act more slowly but have widespread and long-lasting effects.

1. Major Glands and Their Roles

- **Hypothalamus:** The master switchboard in the brain; connects nervous and endocrine systems.

- **Pituitary gland:** The "CEO gland," regulating growth, reproduction, and other glands.
- **Thyroid gland:** Regulates metabolism, energy, and body temperature.
- **Adrenal glands:** Sit atop the kidneys; release adrenaline and cortisol for stress response.
- **Pancreas:** Produces insulin and glucagon to regulate blood sugar.
- **Gonads (ovaries/testes):** Produce sex hormones — estrogen, progesterone, testosterone.
- **Pineal gland:** Produces melatonin, regulating sleep-wake cycles.

2. Hormones as Performance Modulators

Hormones function like software updates or "settings" that adjust your machine:

- **Adrenaline (epinephrine):** Fight-or-flight activation — faster heartbeat, sharper focus.
- **Cortisol:** Manages stress, blood sugar, inflammation. Too much = burnout; too little = fatigue.
- **Insulin & glucagon:** Balance blood sugar (fuel availability).
- **Growth hormone:** Stimulates muscle, bone, and tissue repair.
- **Testosterone & estrogen:** Regulate reproductive functions, muscle growth, mood.
- **Thyroxine (T4) & triiodothyronine (T3):** Control metabolism speed.

3. Performance Ranges

- Hormone levels fluctuate naturally (circadian rhythms, stress, nutrition, aging).
- Example: Cortisol peaks in the morning to wake you up, then declines through the day.
- Example: Melatonin rises in darkness, preparing the brain for sleep.

4. Endocrine Health & Maintenance

- **Nutrition:** Balanced diet with adequate micronutrients (iodine for thyroid, zinc for testosterone).
- **Sleep:** Essential for hormone regulation.
- **Exercise:** Stimulates growth hormone, testosterone, and improves insulin sensitivity.
- **Stress management:** Chronic stress keeps cortisol high, disrupting other hormones.
- **Medical monitoring:** Bloodwork can identify imbalances (thyroid disorders, diabetes, adrenal issues).

The Immune System: Security and Defense

If the endocrine system is software, the immune system is **your firewall and anti-virus software**. It constantly patrols, scans, and neutralizes threats.

1. First Line of Defense: Barriers

- **Skin:** A physical wall, preventing entry of pathogens.
- **Mucous membranes:** Trap particles in airways, digestive tract.
- **Stomach acid:** Destroys microbes in food.

2. Innate Immune System (Rapid Response)

- **White blood cells (phagocytes, natural killer cells):** Attack anything foreign.
- **Inflammation:** Heat, redness, swelling — a rapid alarm and cleanup response.
- **Fever:** Raises body temperature to make conditions hostile for pathogens.

3. Adaptive Immune System (Targeted Defense)

- **Lymphocytes:**
    - *B cells:* Produce antibodies to neutralize specific invaders.
    - *T cells:* Destroy infected cells directly.

- **Memory cells:** Remember past invaders, enabling faster, stronger responses next time. (Why vaccines and natural immunity from prior infection work.)

Immune Communication

The immune system coordinates through chemical signals (cytokines). It's like a security team that not only detects intruders but calls in reinforcements when needed.

Performance Ranges of Defense

- **Response time:** Innate immunity reacts within minutes to hours. Adaptive immunity may take days on first exposure but is lightning-fast on repeat encounters.
- **Capacity:** The immune system faces thousands of daily challenges — from dust particles to pathogens — and neutralizes most without symptoms.
- **Balance matters:** Too weak = infections. Too strong = autoimmune disorders (body attacking itself).

Maintenance of the Control Panel

Endocrine Care

1. **Prioritize consistent sleep:** Critical for melatonin, cortisol, and growth hormone rhythms.
2. **Fuel with balance:** Avoid extreme diets that disrupt blood sugar or hormone production.
3. **Exercise smartly:** Both strength and endurance training improve hormone balance.
4. **Manage stress:** Meditation, breathing, and downtime reduce cortisol load.

Immune Care

1. **Nutrition:**
    - Protein supports antibody production.
    - Vitamins C, D, and zinc strengthen defenses.
    - Probiotics (fermented foods) support gut immunity.
2. **Movement:** Regular moderate activity boosts immune function; extreme overtraining can suppress it.
3. **Hygiene:** Wash hands, but don't live in a sterile bubble — mild exposure trains immunity.

Environmental Factors

- **Stress:** Chronic stress weakens immunity and disrupts endocrine balance.
- **Sleep deprivation:** Reduces immune response and hormone regulation.
- **Nutrition gaps:** Low vitamin D (common in winter) weakens both systems.
- **Toxins/pollutants:** Chemicals and smoking impair immunity and hormone function.

Common Issues & Troubleshooting

- **Diabetes:** Faulty insulin regulation; requires lifestyle management or medication.
- **Thyroid disorders:** Overactive (hyperthyroidism) = jittery, weight loss; underactive (hypothyroidism) = fatigue, weight gain.
- **Autoimmune diseases:** Immune system attacks self (e.g., rheumatoid arthritis, lupus).
- **Allergies:** Immune system overreacts to harmless substances (pollen, dust).
- **Chronic stress syndrome:** Constant cortisol load leading to fatigue, weight gain, and suppressed immunity.

Operating Tips for Your Control Panel

1. **Sleep 7–9 hours per night.**
2. **Eat a nutrient-dense diet:** Protein, vitamins, minerals.
3. **Stay active but avoid chronic overtraining.**
4. **Manage stress intentionally.**
5. **Protect against infection:** Hygiene and avoiding unnecessary exposure when ill.
6. **Listen to your dashboard:** Fatigue, sudden weight changes, frequent illness = check endocrine/immune systems.

Your body's control panel — the endocrine and immune systems — may not be as visible as your muscles or as obvious as your skeleton, but they are the **regulators and guardians** of everything you do. They fine-tune performance, manage stress, fuel adaptation, and stand guard against invaders.

Just like a machine needs regular software updates and reliable security, your body thrives when these systems are respected, supported, and maintained.

Part 3

Maintenance

&

Upgrades

Chapter 10

Fueling the Machine: Nutrition Basics

Fuel for the Engine

Every machine requires fuel. Cars run on gasoline or electricity. Rockets need liquid oxygen and hydrogen. Computers draw electrical current.

Your body, though far more complex, is no different. It needs the right fuel, in the right amounts, at the right time. Too little and performance stalls. Too much of the wrong kind and the system clogs, overheats, or breaks down. Unlike most machines, however, the human body is **fuel-flexible** — it can run on carbohydrates, fats, and proteins in different proportions, switching as needed.

This chapter explains the **basics of nutrition**, breaking down macronutrients, micronutrients, hydration, and the principles of fueling for both daily living and performance. Think of it as the "fuel chapter" in your owner's manual.

The Macronutrients: Your Primary Fuel Sources

1. Carbohydrates – High-Octane Fuel

- **Function:** The body's preferred energy source, especially for the brain and during high-intensity exercise.
- **Storage:** Stored as glycogen in muscles and the liver (~1,500–2,000 kcal max). Once full, excess is stored as fat.
- **Sources:** Whole grains, fruits, vegetables, legumes.
- **Fuel profile:**
    - Quick energy release.

- Critical for sprinting, lifting, and explosive movements.
- Brain relies almost exclusively on glucose under normal conditions.

---

2. Fats – Long-Range Fuel

- **Function:** Concentrated energy source (9 kcal/gram vs. 4 kcal/gram for carbs/protein). Best for endurance and low-intensity activity.
- **Storage:** Virtually unlimited — even lean individuals carry 30,000+ kcal in fat reserves.
- **Sources:** Avocados, nuts, olive oil, fatty fish.
- **Fuel profile:**
  - Slow, steady burn.
  - Essential for hormone production and cell membranes.
  - Primary fuel during rest and long-duration exercise.

---

3. Protein – The Building Blocks

- **Function:** Primary role is repair, maintenance, and building (muscle, enzymes, hormones, immune function). Secondary role as fuel in extreme conditions.
- **Sources:** Lean meats, poultry, fish, dairy, legumes, soy, quinoa.
- **Fuel profile:**
  - 4 kcal/gram.

- Not stored for fuel — muscle is broken down if dietary intake is insufficient.
- Vital for recovery and performance longevity.

---

4. The Fuel Mix

Think of your body like a hybrid engine:

- At **idle/rest:** Mostly fat burning (~70% fat, 30% carb).
- At **moderate activity:** Mix shifts toward carbs (50/50).
- At **high intensity:** Almost all carbs (80–90%).
- During **starvation or low-carb diets:** Protein and fat take over, ketones fuel the brain.

Micronutrients: The Spark Plugs and Lubricants

Macronutrients provide fuel, but **micronutrients** keep the engine running smoothly. They don't supply energy, but they enable every reaction in the body.

1. Vitamins

- **Fat-soluble:** A, D, E, K (stored in fat, risk of excess if oversupplemented).

- **Water-soluble:** B vitamins, C (must be consumed regularly).

Roles:

- Vitamin D = calcium absorption, bone health.
- Vitamin C = collagen synthesis, immune defense.
- B vitamins = energy metabolism.

2. Minerals

- **Calcium:** Bone strength, muscle contraction.
- **Iron:** Oxygen transport in red blood cells.
- **Magnesium:** Nerve function, energy production.
- **Zinc:** Immune function, wound healing.
- **Potassium & sodium:** Fluid balance and nerve signaling.

A deficiency in even one can cause performance breakdowns — like running an engine with faulty spark plugs.

Hydration: The Coolant and Medium

Water is not just a beverage. It's the **coolant, transport medium, and solvent** for nearly every bodily process.

- **Body composition:** ~60% water by weight.
- **Functions:**
    - Regulates temperature (sweat).
    - Transports nutrients in blood plasma.
    - Cushions joints.
    - Supports digestion and waste removal.

Performance ranges:

- Mild dehydration (1–2% body weight lost): Fatigue, reduced endurance, impaired focus.
- Severe dehydration (5%+): Heat illness, dizziness, collapse.

Operating tip: Urine color is your built-in gauge: pale yellow = optimal; dark amber = low fuel.

Principles of Fueling

1. Balance

A balanced mix of carbs, fats, and proteins ensures fuel flexibility. Extreme elimination diets can work short-term but often compromise long-term performance.

2. Timing

- **Before activity:** Carbs + protein (e.g., oatmeal with nuts).

- **During endurance events:** Easily digested carbs every 45–60 minutes.
- **After activity:** Protein + carbs to repair muscle and replenish glycogen.

3. Quality

Not all fuel is equal:

- Whole foods = slow, sustained energy + nutrients.
- Processed foods = quick spikes, crashes, poor maintenance.

4. Individualization

Metabolism varies. Some thrive with higher carbs, others with higher fat intake. Testing and adjusting is key.

Environmental Factors

- **Heat:** Increases water and electrolyte needs.
- **Altitude:** Raises carb requirements (oxygen-efficient fuel).
- **Cold:** Boosts calorie demand to maintain body temperature.
- **Stress & sleep deprivation:** Increase cravings and alter hormone regulation of appetite.

Common Issues & Troubleshooting

- **Energy crashes:** Often due to high-sugar foods followed by insulin spikes.
- **Micronutrient deficiencies:** Fatigue, poor recovery, frequent illness.
- **Overeating:** Clogs the system with excess storage.
- **Undereating:** Leads to muscle breakdown, poor immune defense.
- **Electrolyte imbalance:** Cramps, weakness, irregular heartbeat.

Operating Tips for Nutrition

1. **Eat whole, minimally processed foods most of the time.**
2. **Include protein with every meal.**
3. **Balance carbs and fats for your lifestyle and activity.**
4. **Hydrate consistently — don't wait for thirst.**
5. **Use food as fuel, not just entertainment.**
6. **Check your dashboard:** Fatigue, frequent illness, or poor recovery may be signs of fuel imbalance.

Nutrition is the most direct way you control your body's performance. You can't change your skeleton's design or swap out your nervous system's wiring, but every bite of food and sip of water is a choice about how your machine runs.

The right fuel mix doesn't just power daily life — it builds resilience, sharpens focus, and extends the warranty on your body for decades.

Chapter 11

Performance Upgrades: Exercise & Training

Stress to Strength

Every advanced machine requires testing and upgrades. Cars need performance tuning to run at peak efficiency. Software requires updates to stay fast, secure, and bug-free.

Your body works the same way. The **stress of exercise** is the upgrade trigger. Place the right demands on muscles, bones, heart, lungs, and nervous system, and they adapt — becoming stronger, faster, more efficient. Place no demand, and they regress, losing power and resilience. Place *too much* demand without recovery, and the system breaks down.

Exercise is the single most effective way to upgrade your human machine. This chapter explores the principles of training, the types of fitness adaptations, and how to optimize your personal performance program.

Why Exercise is an Upgrade

1. Structural Upgrades

- **Bones:** Stress increases density (Wolff's Law).
- **Muscles:** Microtears heal stronger.
- **Tendons & ligaments:** Thicken with load, improving resilience.

2. Systemic Upgrades

- **Cardiovascular:** Increases stroke volume, lowers resting heart rate.
- **Respiratory:** Expands lung efficiency.
- **Metabolic:** Improves insulin sensitivity, burns fuel more efficiently.

- **Nervous system:** Enhances motor unit recruitment, coordination, and reflexes.

3. Longevity Upgrades

- Reduces risk of heart disease, diabetes, cancer.
- Preserves mobility and independence with age.
- Boosts mental health, reducing depression and anxiety.

Exercise is not optional maintenance — it's the **master upgrade system**.

The Principles of Training

Think of these as the **rules of the upgrade manual**:

1. **Specificity** – Train what you want to improve. Running boosts endurance; lifting boosts strength.
2. **Progressive overload** – Gradually increase load to force adaptation.
3. **Variation** – Mix intensity, duration, and type to avoid stagnation.
4. **Recovery** – Upgrades occur during rest, not during training.
5. **Reversibility** – Stop training, and gains reverse ("use it or lose it").

The Fitness Domains

Training upgrades happen in several domains, each with its own operating principles.

1. Strength (The Power Upgrade)

- **Definition:** Ability to generate force.
- **Benefits:** Stronger frame, better metabolism, injury prevention.
- **How to train:** Resistance training (weights, bands, bodyweight).
- **Key guidelines:**
    - 2–4 sessions/week.
    - 3–5 sets of 5–12 reps for major muscle groups.
    - Focus on compound movements: squats, deadlifts, presses, pulls.

---

2. Endurance (The Efficiency Upgrade)

- **Definition:** Ability to sustain activity over time.
- **Benefits:** Cardiovascular health, fat burning, stamina.
- **How to train:** Walking, running, cycling, swimming, rowing.
- **Key guidelines:**
    - 150+ minutes/week moderate intensity or 75+ minutes vigorous.
    - Use intervals to improve VO_2 max.

- Long slow distance + shorter high-intensity efforts = best results.

---

3. Mobility & Flexibility (The Range Upgrade)

- **Definition:** Ability to move joints through full range of motion.
- **Benefits:** Prevents stiffness, improves performance, lowers injury risk.
- **How to train:** Stretching, yoga, dynamic warm-ups, joint mobility drills.
- **Key guidelines:**
    - Daily practice of 5–10 minutes.
    - Stretch after activity when tissues are warm.

---

4. Power & Speed (The Explosive Upgrade)

- **Definition:** Ability to apply force quickly.
- **Benefits:** Athleticism, agility, fall prevention as you age.
- **How to train:** Sprinting, plyometrics, Olympic lifts, medicine ball throws.
- **Key guidelines:**
    - Train fresh (not in fatigue).
    - Emphasize quality, not volume.

5. Balance & Stability (The Control Upgrade)

- **Definition:** Ability to maintain posture and coordination under challenge.
- **Benefits:** Injury prevention, athletic efficiency, everyday safety.
- **How to train:** Single-leg exercises, stability ball work, balance boards, Tai Chi.
- **Key guidelines:**
    - Integrate with strength and mobility.
    - Particularly vital for older adults.

Programming the Upgrade

Think of programming as the **software scheduling** of your fitness:

- **Beginners:**
    - Full-body strength workouts 2–3x per week.
    - Cardiovascular training 3–5x per week (mix of moderate and vigorous).
    - Flexibility/mobility daily.
- **Intermediate/advanced:**
    - Split programs (upper/lower, push/pull).
    - Periodization: cycles of building, deloading, and recovery.
    - Sport-specific drills layered in.

- **Lifestyle integration:**
  - Use stairs, walk meetings, active commuting.
  - Movement "snacks" (short bursts of activity) throughout the day.

Environmental and System Factors

- **Heat:** Shortens endurance, requires hydration/electrolytes.
- **Cold:** Stiffens joints, demands longer warm-ups.
- **Altitude:** Limits oxygen — endurance harder, but adaptation improves blood efficiency.
- **Stress & sleep:** Poor recovery = reduced gains, higher injury risk.

Common Issues & Troubleshooting

- **Overtraining:** Fatigue, poor sleep, irritability, frequent illness = too much stress, not enough recovery.
- **Injuries:** Usually from poor form, too much load, or inadequate recovery.
- **Plateaus:** Body adapts — change volume, intensity, or exercise selection.
- **Motivation loss:** Mix in variety, set goals, track progress.

Operating Tips for Exercise & Training

1. **Start where you are, not where you wish you were.**
2. **Consistency beats intensity.** Regular practice matters more than occasional extremes.
3. **Respect form before load.** Quality movement prevents breakdown.
4. **Balance the system.** Train strength, endurance, mobility, stability together.
5. **Schedule recovery.** Rest days are part of the program.
6. **Track progress.** Metrics = feedback = motivation.

Exercise is not punishment. It is the **upgrade protocol** your body needs to grow stronger, faster, and more resilient. Without it, systems decline. With it, every aspect of performance improves — from your bones and muscles to your brain and mood.

Like updating the software and tuning the engine of a high-performance machine, training is how you unlock your body's full potential. The beauty of this system? You can begin at any age, any fitness level, and still see dramatic improvements.

Chapter 12

Recovery Mode: Rest, Sleep, and Regeneration

The Power of Downtime

Every machine requires downtime. Airplanes undergo maintenance between flights. Computers reboot to install updates. High-performance cars overheat without pit stops.

Your body is no different. Training, working, and even daily living create stress — microtears in muscle, strain on joints, depletion of fuel stores, and mental fatigue. **Recovery is where the magic happens.**

This chapter explains why rest and sleep are not luxuries but essential functions, how recovery works on physical and neurological levels, and how to optimize it for performance and longevity.

Why Recovery Matters

1. Repair and Growth

- **Muscles:** Exercise creates microtears; rest repairs them, making fibers thicker and stronger.
- **Bones:** Weight-bearing stress signals remodeling; recovery allows rebuilding.
- **Nervous system:** Downtime recalibrates motor pathways and reaction times.

2. Hormone Regulation

- **Growth hormone & testosterone:** Peak during deep sleep, fueling repair.
- **Cortisol:** Drops at night, reducing stress load.
- **Melatonin:** Signaled in response to darkness and sleep onset, supporting circadian rhythm.

3. Mental Reboot

- **Memory consolidation:** Sleep integrates short-term memories into long-term storage.
- **Emotional regulation:** Adequate rest stabilizes mood, reduces anxiety.
- **Creativity boost:** REM sleep stimulates problem-solving and insight.

Sleep: The Master Recovery Tool

Sleep is the most powerful recovery protocol in your manual. It is not "doing nothing" — it's active regeneration.

1. Sleep Stages

- **Stage 1 (Light sleep):** Transition, easy to wake.
- **Stage 2 (Deeper light sleep):** Brain slows, body relaxes.
- **Stage 3 (Deep sleep):** Tissue repair, hormone release, immune strengthening.
- **REM (Rapid Eye Movement):** Dreaming, brain processing, memory consolidation.

A full cycle lasts **~90 minutes**, repeating 4–6 times per night. Both deep sleep and REM are critical for recovery.

2. Sleep Requirements

- **Adults:** 7–9 hours.
- **Athletes:** 8–10 hours or naps to support training.
- **Sleep debt:** Missing hours accumulates — recovery can't be cheated.

3. Sleep Quality Factors

- **Consistency:** Same bedtime/wake time = stronger circadian rhythm.
- **Environment:** Dark, cool, quiet room.
- **Habits:** Avoid screens/blue light before bed; limit caffeine and alcohol.

Active Recovery

Not all recovery means lying still. **Active recovery** involves light, restorative activity that boosts circulation without stressing the system.

- **Walking:** Flushes out metabolic byproducts.
- **Mobility drills/yoga:** Keep joints lubricated, reduce stiffness.
- **Low-intensity cardio:** Swimming, cycling at easy pace.
- **Breathing/meditation:** Calms nervous system, lowers stress hormones.

Nutrition for Recovery

Fuel choices directly impact regeneration.

- **Protein:** Supplies amino acids to rebuild muscle.
- **Carbohydrates:** Replenish glycogen stores for next performance cycle.
- **Healthy fats:** Reduce inflammation, support hormone balance.
- **Micronutrients:** Magnesium (relaxation, sleep quality), zinc (healing), vitamin C (tissue repair).
- **Hydration:** Restores fluid balance lost in sweat and respiration.

Recovery Timeframes

Different systems recover at different speeds:

- **Muscles:** 24–72 hours depending on intensity.
- **Nervous system:** May take longer after maximal lifts or high-skill training.
- **Energy systems:** Glycogen stores replenish in 24–48 hours with proper nutrition.
- **Injuries:** Microtears = days; serious strains or breaks = weeks to months.

Stress and Recovery Balance

Recovery is not just physical — it's about balancing **stress and rest**.

- **Sympathetic nervous system (fight or flight):** Training, work, stress.
- **Parasympathetic nervous system (rest and digest):** Sleep, recovery, calm states.

Too much sympathetic activity without parasympathetic balance leads to **burnout** — fatigue, poor performance, illness.

Tools and Strategies for Recovery

1. Sleep Hygiene Checklist

- Regular bedtime.
- Dark, cool, quiet room.
- Limit caffeine after midday.
- Screens off 60 minutes before bed.
- Evening wind-down ritual (reading, stretching).

2. Physical Recovery Tools

- **Stretching & mobility:** Reduce stiffness.
- **Massage/foam rolling:** Increase circulation, relieve tension.

- **Contrast therapy (hot/cold):** Stimulate blood flow, reduce inflammation.
- **Compression gear:** Assists venous return, speeds recovery.

3. Mind-Body Recovery

- Meditation, journaling, or gratitude practices reduce stress.
- Breathwork (slow diaphragmatic breathing) activates parasympathetic mode.
- Social connection and laughter = underrated but powerful recovery boosters.

Common Issues & Troubleshooting

- **Insomnia:** Difficulty falling or staying asleep. Often tied to stress, caffeine, or screen use.
- **Overtraining syndrome:** Chronic fatigue, irritability, elevated resting heart rate.
- **Poor recovery nutrition:** Skipping post-training fuel slows adaptation.
- **Stress overload:** Work + training + life stress with no downtime = guaranteed breakdown.

Operating Tips for Recovery Mode

1. **Sleep is non-negotiable.** Build your day around it.
2. **Use active recovery.** Gentle movement accelerates healing.
3. **Fuel the rebuild.** Protein + carbs after exercise.
4. **Hydrate before, during, after training.**
5. **Balance stress and calm.** Build parasympathetic activities into your day.
6. **Listen to your dashboard.** Persistent soreness, fatigue, or irritability = extend recovery.

Recovery is the **installation phase of your upgrades**. Training, work, and stress load the system, but adaptation and progress only occur if you shut down, recharge, and give the body time to rebuild.

Sleep, rest, and regeneration are not indulgences. They are the foundation of resilience, health, and performance. Treat them as essential maintenance, and your machine will run smoothly for years.

Chapter 13

Routine Service Schedule

Preventive Maintenance

Every machine has a maintenance schedule. Cars need oil changes, tire rotations, and inspections at set mileage intervals. Airplanes require detailed service logs before every flight.

The human body is no different. While it is self-repairing and remarkably durable, it still benefits from **regular maintenance checks** — preventive care, daily habits, and professional screenings that catch problems before they become breakdowns.

In this chapter, we'll lay out a **service schedule for your body**: what to do daily, weekly, monthly, and yearly to keep the system tuned, safe, and performing at its best.

Daily Service Checks

1. Fuel & Hydration

- Eat balanced meals: protein, healthy fats, complex carbs, micronutrients.
- Drink water throughout the day — don't wait for thirst.
- Use the "urine color test" to gauge hydration.

2. Movement

- Minimum: 30 minutes of activity (walking, mobility drills, stretching).
- Avoid long sedentary periods — move every hour.
- Check posture while sitting, standing, and lifting.

3. Sleep & Recovery

- Aim for 7–9 hours of quality sleep.
- Wind down with a consistent bedtime ritual.

- Monitor morning energy: do you wake rested or groggy?

4. Dashboard Scan

Take 60 seconds to check in:

- Any unusual pain?
- Persistent fatigue?
- Mood or focus changes?
- These are early warning lights.

Weekly Service Checks

1. Structured Training

- Strength train 2–3 times.
- Cardio sessions 3–5 times.
- Mobility/flexibility every day (5–10 minutes).

2. Nutrition Audit

- Check your food balance. Too much processed food? Not enough fruits/veggies?
- Ensure adequate protein intake (~0.7–1 g per pound of bodyweight if active).
- Plan meals to avoid relying on convenience fuel.

3. Rest Days

- At least 1–2 active recovery days.
- Walk, stretch, or do yoga instead of intense training.

4. Stress Check

- Journal, meditate, or reflect on your stress levels.
- If stress remains high for multiple weeks, adjust workload or recovery.

Monthly Service Checks

1. Body Composition & Metrics

- Track weight, waist circumference, and strength/fitness progress.
- Note trends, not single-day changes.

2. Mobility & Flexibility Test

- Can you touch your toes?
- Squat to full depth comfortably?
- Rotate shoulders without restriction?

3. Resting Heart Rate

- Take morning pulse before getting up. Rising trends over weeks may indicate fatigue, overtraining, or illness.

4. Personal Maintenance

- Schedule recovery sessions (massage, physiotherapy if needed).
- Rotate workout styles to avoid plateaus.

Annual Service Checks

Like cars needing yearly inspections, your body benefits from professional evaluation:

1. Medical Exam

- Comprehensive physical.
- Blood pressure, cholesterol, blood sugar levels.
- BMI and waist circumference (contextual, not absolute).

2. Blood Work

- CBC (complete blood count).
- Vitamin D, iron, thyroid function (common issues).

- Hormone panel if symptomatic (fatigue, mood swings, unexplained weight change).

3. Preventive Screenings

- Dental check-up (every 6 months).
- Eye exam (every 1–2 years).
- Skin checks (for moles, changes).
- Colon, prostate, breast, or cervical screenings as age/guidelines suggest.

4. Fitness Test

- VO_2 max estimate (cardio efficiency).
- 1-rep strength test or endurance equivalent.
- Mobility and posture assessment.

Lifespan Service Considerations

1. In Your 20s–30s

- Build habits. Peak bone mass, muscle, and cardiovascular capacity are set now.
- Preventive screenings: blood work baseline.

2. In Your 40s–50s

- Prioritize strength training to offset muscle loss.

- Screenings: cholesterol, blood pressure, cancer checks become more critical.

3. In Your 60s and Beyond

- Focus on balance and stability to prevent falls.
- Strength preservation = independence.
- Screen for osteoporosis, diabetes, and cognitive health.

Common Issues & Troubleshooting

- **Ignoring warning lights:** Small pains become chronic injuries if unchecked.
- **Skipping service checks:** Preventive care catches problems early; neglect often means expensive repairs later.
- **Lifestyle imbalance:** Poor sleep, excess stress, or bad fuel can undo even good exercise habits.
- **Procrastination:** Maintenance delayed is performance denied.

Operating Tips for Routine Service

1. **Think preventive, not reactive.** Don't wait for breakdowns.
2. **Track metrics, not just feelings.** Data gives objective insight.
3. **Schedule professional check-ups annually.**
4. **Integrate daily and weekly maintenance.** Small actions compound over years.
5. **Respect age and stage.** Adjust service schedule as your machine ages.
6. **Customize.** Every body is unique — tailor fuel, training, and recovery to your system.

Machines fail when neglected. They thrive with maintenance. The human body is the same — but with one incredible advantage: it adapts, improves, and grows stronger with the right service routine.

Daily, weekly, monthly, and yearly maintenance isn't restrictive. It's liberating. It ensures your body operates at full potential, avoids costly breakdowns, and performs beautifully well into old age.

Part 4

Troubleshooting

&

Repairs

Chapter 14

Warning Lights: Symptoms You Shouldn't Ignore

The Dashboard of the Human Machine

Every vehicle has dashboard lights — indicators that alert the driver to fuel levels, oil pressure, or engine trouble. Smart drivers don't ignore these signals. A blinking oil light might mean a minor issue today, but left unchecked, it could destroy the engine tomorrow.

Your body has its own dashboard. Unlike cars, it doesn't come with a digital readout or manual explaining each signal. Instead, it communicates through **symptoms**: pain, fatigue, changes in appetite, altered sleep, skin changes, or unusual sensations.

This chapter is about learning to **read those warning lights** — distinguishing between normal, temporary fluctuations and signals that require immediate attention.

The Philosophy of Symptoms

1. Pain as a Signal, Not an Enemy

Pain isn't the problem itself — it's a **message**. Treating pain with only medication is like covering your car's "check engine" light with tape. You may feel better, but the underlying issue remains.

2. Acute vs. Chronic Signals

- **Acute:** Sudden, sharp signals (e.g., sprained ankle). Often protective.
- **Chronic:** Persistent, low-level signals (e.g., back pain for months). Often indicate wear, imbalance, or deeper issues.

3. Listening Early Saves Repairs

Catching problems at the "blinking light" stage is easier than waiting for total breakdown.

Symptoms You Should Never Ignore

Here are the "red lights" on your dashboard — indicators that should not be dismissed.

1. Chest Pain or Pressure

- May signal heart attack, angina, or vascular issues.
- Especially concerning if paired with shortness of breath, sweating, or radiating pain in arm/jaw.
- **Action:** Immediate medical attention.

2. Sudden Severe Headache

- Could signal aneurysm, stroke, or high blood pressure crisis.
- **Action:** Emergency care if worst-ever pain or accompanied by confusion/vision loss.

3. Unexplained Weight Loss

- Losing >5% body weight in a month without trying may indicate metabolic, hormonal, or cancer-related issues.
- **Action:** Medical evaluation.

4. Persistent Fever

- Ongoing temperature above 100.4°F (38°C) without clear cause = infection or inflammation.
- **Action:** Rule out chronic infection or autoimmune disease.

5. Shortness of Breath

- If not explained by exertion, may signal asthma, infection, blood clot, or heart issue.
- **Action:** Medical evaluation, especially if sudden.

6. Unusual Bleeding or Bruising

- Could mean clotting disorder, vitamin deficiency, or cancer.
- **Action:** Seek medical testing.

7. Numbness or Weakness

- Especially one-sided weakness, facial droop, or slurred speech = possible stroke.
- **Action:** Emergency response (time-sensitive).

8. Persistent Digestive Changes

- Ongoing diarrhea, constipation, or blood in stool may indicate GI disease or cancer.
- **Action:** Medical consultation.

9. Night Sweats or Persistent Fatigue

- Could signal infection, hormonal imbalance, or cancer.
- **Action:** Professional evaluation.

10. Sudden Vision or Hearing Changes

- Warning sign of stroke, vascular issues, or neurological disease.
- **Action:** Urgent care.

Yellow Lights: Cautionary Symptoms

Not all signals mean "pull over immediately," but they require monitoring and often lifestyle adjustments.

- **Joint aches/stiffness:** May be overtraining, poor form, or early arthritis.
- **Frequent colds/illness:** Suggests stress or immune suppression.

- **Sleep disturbances:** Can stem from stress, screen use, caffeine, or deeper hormonal imbalance.
- **Mood changes:** Irritability, anxiety, or depression may indicate overtraining, poor nutrition, or underlying conditions.
- **Skin changes:** Rashes, slow-healing wounds, or new moles = dermatology check.

These are "service soon" warnings — don't panic, but don't ignore.

Self-Monitoring Tools

Think of these as your **home diagnostics kit**:

1. Resting Heart Rate

- Take pulse upon waking. Normal = 60–100 bpm. Athletes = 30–50.
- Rising trend = fatigue, overtraining, or illness.

2. Blood Pressure

- Ideal = ~120/80. Persistent >140/90 = service check needed.

3. Sleep Quality

- Track total hours and whether you wake refreshed.

- Chronic poor sleep is a warning light.

4. Energy Levels

- Rate daily energy 1–10. Persistent <5 = imbalance.

5. Pain Journal

- Record type, intensity, triggers. Patterns reveal causes.

When to Seek Help

It's tempting to ignore symptoms until they interfere with daily life. But like machines, **small problems compound**.

- **Immediate help:** Red light symptoms (chest pain, severe headache, weakness, bleeding).
- **Professional check:** Persistent yellow light symptoms (fatigue, joint pain, mood changes).
- **Self-adjustment:** Mild, temporary issues that respond to rest, recovery, or better fuel.

Rule of thumb: **If something feels "off" for more than two weeks, investigate.**

Common Mistakes in Reading Warning Lights

- **Ignoring pain:** Treating it as weakness instead of feedback.
- **Masking with meds:** Painkillers hide signals but don't fix causes.
- **Over-Googling:** Self-diagnosis without professional input often causes anxiety.
- **Normalizing dysfunction:** "I'm always tired," "My knees always hurt" = not normal, just common.

Operating Tips for Dashboard Monitoring

1. **Pay attention early.** The sooner you act, the easier the fix.
2. **Track data.** Numbers reveal trends, symptoms alone don't.
3. **Balance judgment.** Don't panic over every ache, but don't ignore persistent red flags.
4. **Use professional help.** Mechanics fix cars; doctors help humans.
5. **Don't normalize breakdowns.** Common $\neq$ healthy.

Your body is equipped with one of the most sophisticated diagnostic dashboards in existence. Pain, fatigue, mood, appetite, sleep, and other signals aren't nuisances — they're **warning lights designed to protect you**.

Learning to read those signals, respond appropriately, and seek help when needed is one of the most valuable skills you can develop. Machines break without warning when ignored. Your body, however, almost always tells you first — if you're willing to listen.

Chapter 15

Common Breakdowns & Fixes

Field Repairs for the Human Machine

Even the best-maintained machines encounter breakdowns. Cars get flat tires, planes experience turbulence, computers crash. Your body, too, experiences malfunctions — sprains, strains, fatigue, colds, or digestive issues.

Most breakdowns are **not catastrophic**. With the right knowledge, you can often troubleshoot and repair them before they escalate. This chapter covers the most common physical and functional issues people face, how to handle them, and when to call in professional mechanics (a.k.a. doctors and therapists).

Musculoskeletal Breakdowns

1. Sprains (Ligaments)

- **Cause:** Overstretching or tearing ligaments (e.g., ankle twist).
- **Symptoms:** Pain, swelling, bruising, instability.
- **Fix:**
    - RICE protocol: **R**est, **I**ce, **C**ompression, **E**levation (first 48 hours).
    - Gradual mobility restoration.
    - Physical therapy if severe.
- **When to seek help:** Inability to bear weight, suspected fracture.

---

2. Strains (Muscles/Tendons)

- **Cause:** Overstretching or tearing muscle fibers/tendons (e.g., hamstring pull).
- **Symptoms:** Sharp pain, weakness, swelling.

- **Fix:**
    - RICE protocol initially.
    - Gentle stretching after acute phase.
    - Gradual strengthening program.
- **When to seek help:** Severe weakness or visible muscle deformity.

---

3. Tendinitis

- **Cause:** Overuse injury of tendons (e.g., tennis elbow, runner's knee).
- **Symptoms:** Localized pain, tenderness with movement.
- **Fix:**
    - Relative rest (reduce, not eliminate activity).
    - Ice, anti-inflammatory strategies.
    - Eccentric strengthening exercises.
- **When to seek help:** Pain persisting >4–6 weeks.

---

4. Back Pain

- **Cause:** Poor posture, lifting mechanics, weak core, disc issues.
- **Symptoms:** Ache, stiffness, radiating leg pain (sciatica).

- **Fix:**
    - Core strengthening, posture correction.
    - Heat therapy for stiffness, ice for acute inflammation.
    - Movement > bed rest.
- **When to seek help:** Numbness, bowel/bladder changes, severe radiating pain.

Fatigue & Energy Breakdowns

1. General Fatigue

- **Cause:** Poor sleep, stress, overtraining, under-fueling.
- **Fix:**
    - Check sleep hygiene.
    - Ensure balanced nutrition and hydration.
    - Reduce training volume temporarily.
- **When to seek help:** Fatigue lasting >2 weeks despite lifestyle fixes.

---

2. Overtraining Syndrome

- **Cause:** Too much exercise, not enough recovery.

- **Symptoms:** Declining performance, irritability, insomnia, elevated resting heart rate.
- **Fix:**
    o Rest (days to weeks).
    o Reduce volume/intensity long term.
    o Incorporate parasympathetic activities (yoga, meditation).
- **When to seek help:** Persistent symptoms despite rest.

---

3. Burnout

- **Cause:** Chronic stress (work + training + life load).
- **Symptoms:** Mental exhaustion, loss of motivation, emotional flatness.
- **Fix:**
    o Prioritize sleep.
    o Reduce obligations temporarily.
    o Add restorative practices (nature time, hobbies, social connection).
- **When to seek help:** Severe depression, inability to function.

Illness & Immune Breakdowns

1. Common Cold

- **Cause:** Viral infection.
- **Symptoms:** Congestion, sore throat, fatigue, mild fever.
- **Fix:**
    - Rest, hydration, symptom relief (steam, honey, saline sprays).
    - Resume activity gradually.
- **When to seek help:** Fever >102°F, symptoms >10 days, severe chest pain.

---

2. Flu

- **Cause:** Influenza virus.
- **Symptoms:** High fever, chills, body aches, cough, fatigue.
- **Fix:**
    - Rest, fluids, antivirals (if prescribed early).
    - Avoid exercise until fully recovered.
- **When to seek help:** Shortness of breath, chest pain, worsening after initial improvement.

---

3. Food Poisoning / GI Upset

- **Cause:** Contaminated food/water.

- **Symptoms:** Vomiting, diarrhea, cramps, dehydration.
- **Fix:**
    - Hydration with electrolytes.
    - Bland foods (rice, bananas, toast) once stable.
- **When to seek help:** Blood in stool, dehydration signs, illness lasting >3 days.

---

4. Allergic Reactions

- **Cause:** Immune system overreaction (food, pollen, insect bites).
- **Symptoms:** Hives, swelling, difficulty breathing (in severe cases).
- **Fix:**
    - Antihistamines for mild reactions.
    - Epinephrine and emergency care for anaphylaxis.
- **When to seek help:** Always for severe reactions.

Hydration & Electrolyte Breakdowns

1. Dehydration

- **Symptoms:** Thirst, dark urine, fatigue, headache, dizziness.
- **Fix:** Drink water steadily; add electrolytes if sweating heavily.

2. Heat Exhaustion / Heat Stroke

- **Symptoms:** Dizziness, nausea, confusion, high body temp.
- **Fix:** Cool environment, fluids, ice packs.
- **When to seek help:** Heat stroke (confusion, fainting, no sweating) = medical emergency.

3. Electrolyte Imbalance

- **Symptoms:** Muscle cramps, irregular heartbeat, weakness.
- **Fix:** Balanced hydration with sodium, potassium, magnesium.

Skin & Minor Surface Breakdowns

1. Cuts & Scrapes

- **Fix:** Clean, disinfect, bandage.
- **When to seek help:** Deep wounds, signs of infection.

2. Blisters

- **Cause:** Friction (shoes, tools).
- **Fix:** Keep clean, avoid popping unless necessary, cover with padding.

3. Sunburn

- **Cause:** Excess UV exposure.
- **Fix:** Aloe, hydration, cool compresses.
- **Prevention:** Sunscreen, protective clothing.

Recovery Timelines

Approximate timelines for common issues:

- **Mild strain/sprain:** 1–3 weeks.
- **Moderate strain/sprain:** 4–6 weeks.
- **Tendinitis:** 6–12 weeks (with rehab).
- **Colds:** 7–10 days.
- **Flu:** 1–2 weeks.

- **Minor cuts/scrapes:** 1–2 weeks.
- **Burnout/fatigue:** Variable — weeks to months depending on severity.

Operating Tips for Everyday Breakdowns

1. **Don't panic.** Most breakdowns are routine and repairable.
2. **Listen to pain.** Sharp, sudden pain = stop and assess.
3. **Respect rest.** Pushing through often worsens damage.
4. **Use RICE.** First-line care for most musculoskeletal injuries.
5. **Stay hydrated and fueled.** Many minor issues trace back to low fluids or poor nutrition.
6. **Know red flags.** Severe chest pain, sudden weakness, uncontrollable bleeding = emergency.

Breakdowns happen — even in well-maintained machines. The difference between temporary downtime and catastrophic failure is **awareness and timely repair**. Most sprains, strains, colds, and fatigue episodes are minor if addressed early and given proper recovery.

The goal isn't to avoid all breakdowns — that's impossible. The goal is to become a skilled operator of your machine, able to troubleshoot, apply the right fixes, and return to performance safely.

Chapter 16

Software Errors: Mental & Emotional Health

The Software Layer

Even the most powerful hardware — processors, memory, wiring — is useless if the software crashes. A computer with corrupted code freezes, a plane's navigation system fails without reliable programming, and a car's onboard computer can render the engine useless despite perfect mechanics.

Your body is no different. The **mind is the software**. It interprets, directs, and integrates every physical process. When mental or emotional health suffers, performance suffers — even if the frame, engine, wiring, and power supply are perfectly maintained.

This chapter explores the fundamentals of mental and emotional well-being, the warning signs of "software errors," and practical strategies for keeping your inner operating system running smoothly.

Why Mental & Emotional Health Matters

1. The Mind–Body Connection

- Stress can raise blood pressure, disrupt digestion, and weaken immunity.
- Anxiety and depression affect energy, sleep, appetite, and motivation.
- Positive emotional states improve performance, resilience, and longevity.

2. Performance Dependence

Mental health determines:

- **Focus & decision-making.**
- **Stress response.**
- **Consistency in training, nutrition, and recovery.**

A healthy body without a healthy mind is like a car with a full tank of gas but no driver.

Common Software Errors

1. Stress Overload

- **Symptoms:** Irritability, sleep problems, digestive upset, headaches.
- **Cause:** Chronic activation of sympathetic nervous system (fight/flight).
- **Impact:** Elevated cortisol, suppressed immunity, burnout risk.

2. Anxiety

- **Symptoms:** Restlessness, racing thoughts, muscle tension, rapid heartbeat.
- **Cause:** Overactive threat detection system.
- **Impact:** Impaired performance, reduced focus, exhaustion.

3. Depression

- **Symptoms:** Persistent sadness, lack of motivation, fatigue, appetite/sleep changes.
- **Cause:** Multifactorial (neurochemical imbalance, life stress, trauma).
- **Impact:** Reduced engagement, slowed recovery, impaired health behaviors.

4. Burnout

- **Symptoms:** Emotional exhaustion, detachment, reduced accomplishment.
- **Cause:** Chronic stress without adequate recovery.
- **Impact:** Decline in both mental and physical performance.

5. Cognitive Decline / Brain Fog

- **Symptoms:** Poor focus, forgetfulness, reduced mental clarity.
- **Cause:** Sleep deprivation, poor nutrition, chronic stress, illness.
- **Impact:** Impaired decision-making, reduced productivity.

Warning Lights in Mental Health

Just like dashboard indicators, your mind sends signals:

- Persistent fatigue despite sleep.
- Loss of interest in activities.
- Difficulty concentrating.
- Social withdrawal.
- Sudden mood swings.
- Changes in appetite or weight.
- Thoughts of self-harm (critical red light).

Rule of thumb: If mental or emotional symptoms last more than **two weeks** or interfere with daily function, professional help is warranted.

Maintenance for Mental & Emotional Health

1. Sleep Hygiene

- Regular sleep improves emotional regulation and cognitive performance.
- Sleep deprivation worsens mood and anxiety.

2. Stress Management

- **Breathing techniques:** Slow diaphragmatic breathing activates parasympathetic system.

- **Mindfulness & meditation:** Reduce rumination and improve focus.
- **Nature exposure:** Walks outdoors lower cortisol and boost mood.

3. Social Connection

- Strong relationships protect against depression and anxiety.
- Isolation is as damaging as smoking to long-term health.

4. Nutrition

- Omega-3s, B-vitamins, magnesium, and antioxidants support brain health.
- Blood sugar stability prevents mood swings.

5. Physical Activity

- Exercise releases endorphins and serotonin.
- Regular activity reduces depression risk by up to 30–40%.

Software Updates: Mental Training

Just as athletes train their bodies, mental training upgrades emotional resilience.

- **Visualization:** Mental rehearsal improves performance.
- **Goal setting:** Clear, measurable goals improve motivation.
- **Gratitude journaling:** Rewires focus toward positives, reducing stress.
- **Cognitive reframing:** Shifting perspective changes emotional impact.

Environmental Factors

- **Workload:** Excessive demands without recovery fuel burnout.
- **Digital overload:** Constant notifications and screen time fragment attention.
- **Substances:** Alcohol, caffeine, and drugs can disrupt mental balance.
- **Environment:** Light, noise, and clutter affect mood and productivity.

Common Fixes & When to Seek Help

Self-Service Fixes

- Sleep optimization, exercise, nutrition, mindfulness.

- Social connection, hobbies, downtime.

Professional Tune-Ups

- Therapy or counseling (CBT, talk therapy, etc.).
- Medical evaluation for persistent depression, anxiety, or cognitive changes.
- Medication if indicated, under professional supervision.

Emergency Warning

- **Thoughts of self-harm or suicide** = critical error.
- **Immediate action:** Reach out to a professional, crisis hotline, or emergency services. This is not a "wait and see" issue.

Operating Tips for Mental & Emotional Health

1. **Schedule downtime.** Recovery isn't just physical.
2. **Limit digital noise.** Protect attention span.
3. **Move daily.** Even light activity improves mood.
4. **Fuel your brain.** Prioritize whole foods, omega-3s, and hydration.

5. **Train mental skills.** Mindfulness, visualization, journaling.
6. **Seek connection.** Regularly spend time with people who uplift you.
7. **Don't ignore red lights.** Professional help is maintenance, not weakness.

Your body's hardware can be flawless, but without stable software, performance fails. Mental and emotional health are the unseen drivers of every decision, movement, and relationship.

When the software runs smoothly, you think clearly, feel resilient, and operate at your best. When it glitches, every part of the system suffers. The good news? Mental health, like physical health, responds to training, fuel, rest, and professional support when needed.

Chapter 17

Emergency Repairs: What to Do When Things Go Wrong

Crisis Mode

Even the best-maintained machines encounter emergencies. Cars blow a tire on the highway, computers crash during an important presentation, planes encounter turbulence that requires immediate corrective action.

For the human body, emergencies are inevitable: a fall, a cut, a sudden illness, an accident. In these moments, your ability to respond quickly and appropriately determines whether the outcome is a **minor repair** or a **catastrophic breakdown**.

This chapter outlines **first-response protocols** — what to do immediately when things go wrong — and when to escalate to professional emergency services. Think of it as your quick-access troubleshooting guide.

The Philosophy of First Response

1. Keep Calm

Panic wastes energy and clouds judgment. Calm assessment is step one.

2. Safety First

Before helping, ensure the environment is safe (traffic, fire, electrical hazards). You can't repair a system if you become the next casualty.

3. The "ABC" Framework

In true emergencies, always check in this order:

- **A – Airway:** Is it clear?
- **B – Breathing:** Are they breathing?
- **C – Circulation:** Is there a pulse or severe bleeding?

Common Emergencies & Quick Fixes

1. Severe Bleeding

- **Signs:** Bright red spurting blood (arterial) or steady flow (venous).
- **Immediate Action:**
    - Apply firm, direct pressure with clean cloth/bandage.
    - Elevate limb if possible.
    - Tourniquet may be necessary for controlling arterial bleeding.
- **When to escalate:** Always — uncontrolled bleeding = life-threatening.

2. Choking

- **Signs:** Unable to speak, high-pitched wheeze, grasping throat.
- **Immediate Action:**
    o   Encourage coughing if partial obstruction.
    o   If fully obstructed: Heimlich maneuver (abdominal thrusts).
    o   If unresponsive: Begin CPR.
- **When to escalate:** Always call emergency services if obstruction persists.

---

3. Heart Attack

- **Signs:** Chest pain/pressure, pain radiating to arm/jaw, sweating, nausea.
- **Immediate Action:**
    o   Call emergency services.
    o   Have person chew 325 mg aspirin (if not allergic).
    o   Keep calm and still until help arrives.
- **When to escalate:** Immediately — every minute counts.

---

4. Stroke

- **Signs:** Use **FAST**:
    o   *Face droop,*
    o   *Arm weakness,*

- o *Speech difficulty,*
- o *Time to call emergency services.*
- **Immediate Action:**
  - o Call for emergency help immediately.
  - o Keep person safe and still.
- **When to escalate:** Always — time-sensitive clot treatment may save function.

---

5. Unconsciousness / Fainting

- **Cause:** Temporary drop in blood flow to brain (often harmless, sometimes serious).
- **Immediate Action:**
  - o Lay person flat, elevate legs.
  - o Loosen tight clothing.
  - o Check airway and breathing.
- **When to escalate:** If unconsciousness lasts >1 minute or recurs frequently.

---

6. Seizures

- **Signs:** Sudden convulsions, loss of control.
- **Immediate Action:**
  - o Clear area of sharp objects.
  - o Do not restrain or place anything in mouth.
  - o Place on side after seizure ends (recovery position).
- **When to escalate:** First-time seizure, seizure lasting >5 minutes, or repeated seizures.

7. Burns

- **First-degree:** Red skin, mild pain. Cool under water, aloe.
- **Second-degree:** Blisters, deeper pain. Cool gently, cover with sterile dressing.
- **Third-degree:** White/charred skin, nerve damage. Emergency care required.

Rule: If burns cover face, genitals, hands, feet, or large areas, seek professional help.

---

8. Broken Bones

- **Signs:** Visible deformity, swelling, inability to move limb.
- **Immediate Action:**
    - Immobilize with splint.
    - Apply ice to reduce swelling.
    - Do not attempt to reset bone.
- **When to escalate:** Always — requires medical imaging and treatment.

---

9. Heat Illness

- **Heat exhaustion:** Dizziness, heavy sweating, nausea. Move to cool place, hydrate.
- **Heat stroke:** Confusion, hot dry skin, possible unconsciousness.

- Emergency! Cool rapidly (ice packs, cold water), call for help.

---

10. Hypothermia

- **Signs:** Shivering, slurred speech, confusion.
- **Immediate Action:**
    - Warm gradually with blankets, warm drinks.
    - Avoid direct heat (can shock system).
- **When to escalate:** Severe confusion, unconsciousness.

---

11. Allergic Reactions

- **Mild:** Hives, itching. Use antihistamines.
- **Severe (anaphylaxis):** Difficulty breathing, swelling, rapid drop in blood pressure.
    - Use epinephrine auto-injector if available.
    - Call emergency services immediately.

The Emergency Toolkit

Every operator should keep a **basic first-aid kit** — your toolbox for quick repairs:

- Bandages, gauze, adhesive tape.
- Antiseptic wipes, antibiotic ointment.
- Elastic bandage for sprains.
- Ice packs (instant).
- Gloves and CPR mask.
- Pain relievers (acetaminophen, ibuprofen).
- Antihistamines.
- Epinephrine auto-injector (if prescribed).

Bonus tools: flashlight, emergency contact list, extra water.

Training Your Emergency Response

Knowledge is power. Like learning how to change a tire before you're stranded, learning emergency response skills prepares you for when things go wrong.

- **CPR certification:** Saves lives in cardiac arrest.
- **First aid training:** Basic wound care, splints, bleeding control.
- **AED use (defibrillator):** Now common in public places, easy to learn.

When to Call for Professional Mechanics

The golden rule: **If you're unsure, escalate.** Unlike cars, you don't get replacement parts for most body systems.

Call emergency services when:

- Breathing or heartbeat stops.
- Severe bleeding doesn't stop with pressure.
- Sudden neurological changes (weakness, slurred speech).
- Severe chest pain.
- Unconsciousness that lasts >1 minute.
- Severe burns, fractures, or allergic reactions.

Operating Tips for Crisis Situations

1. **Stay calm and assess.** Panic creates more damage.
2. **Check ABCs first.** Airway, breathing, circulation.
3. **Stop major bleeding.** Pressure is your best tool.
4. **Don't overdo fixes.** Support, stabilize, and hand off to professionals.

5. **Learn first aid & CPR.** The best repair is preparation.
6. **Keep a toolkit.** A stocked first-aid kit saves precious time.

Emergencies are inevitable — but disasters are often preventable with the right immediate actions. You don't need to be a surgeon to save a life or prevent further harm. You just need to know the basics, stay calm, and act decisively.

Your body, like any advanced machine, is built to survive challenges — but the operator's response determines whether a breakdown is temporary or permanent.

Part 5

Optimization

&

Longevity

Chapter 18

Performance Tuning: Lifestyle Habits for Longevity

Fine-Tuning the Machine

Every high-performance machine comes with settings you can adjust for better efficiency and durability. Cars can be tuned for better mileage or horsepower. Computers can be optimized with clean software and cooling systems. Airplanes undergo constant adjustments to extend flight hours.

Your body is the same. It's already engineered for longevity — with the right care, many systems can run smoothly well into your 70s, 80s, and beyond. But just like any machine, misuse or neglect accelerates breakdowns, while fine-tuning habits preserve function and extend lifespan.

This chapter explores the **everyday habits** that act as long-term performance tuning knobs: nutrition, movement, recovery, mindset, and environment.

The Longevity Mindset

1. Healthspan vs. Lifespan

- **Lifespan:** How long you live.
- **Healthspan:** How long you live *well*, with independence and vitality.
  Performance tuning aims to extend healthspan — keeping your "engine smooth" rather than just running longer.

2. Compound Interest of Habits

Small daily actions compound over years:

- 20 minutes of walking daily = thousands of extra miles of circulation.

- 10 minutes of stretching daily = decades of preserved mobility.
- Regular sleep = decades of sharper memory and lower disease risk.

Your habits today are deposits in your future health bank.

Fueling for Longevity

1. Balanced Nutrition

- Prioritize **whole foods** over ultra-processed.
- Aim for **variety of colors** on your plate (phytonutrients).
- Balance macronutrients — don't fear carbs, fats, or proteins, but choose quality sources.

2. Caloric Balance

- Chronic overeating accelerates wear (obesity, diabetes, joint stress).
- Caloric moderation and awareness extend system durability.

3. Anti-Inflammatory Diet

- Include omega-3 fats (fish, nuts, seeds).
- Emphasize fruits, vegetables, legumes.
- Limit processed sugars, trans fats.

4. Hydration

Water is not just coolant; it's lubrication, transport, and repair medium. Aim for steady hydration throughout the day.

Movement as Maintenance

1. Daily Activity

- The body thrives on motion.
- Walk, climb stairs, stretch, squat, carry — natural, functional patterns.

2. Structured Exercise

- **Strength training:** 2–3x per week for bone density and muscle preservation.
- **Cardio:** 3–5x per week for cardiovascular endurance.
- **Mobility training:** Daily, to preserve range of motion.

3. Sedentary Risk

- "Sitting disease" accelerates breakdowns (poor circulation, weak posture).
- Use micro-breaks, standing desks, movement snacks.

Recovery as Renewal

1. Sleep

- Prioritize 7–9 hours.
- Protect circadian rhythm with consistent bedtime/wake time.

2. Stress Management

- Chronic stress corrodes systems like rust.
- Breathing practices, mindfulness, and downtime keep stress in balance.

3. Cycles of Effort and Rest

Just as engines overheat if pushed nonstop, your body needs periods of recovery between stress loads.

Environment as a Silent Influence

1. Air Quality

- Clean air = reduced respiratory wear. Avoid smoking/vaping.
- Ventilate indoor spaces, use filters if needed.

2. Light Exposure

- Morning sunlight resets circadian rhythm.

- Limit blue light at night to preserve melatonin cycles.

3. Temperature

- Occasional hormetic stress (cold exposure, heat exposure) builds resilience.

4. Social Environment

- Surround yourself with supportive people.
- Strong relationships are a top predictor of long life.

Mental Habits for Longevity

1. Purpose & Meaning

- Having a "why" drives resilience.
- People with strong life purpose live longer, healthier lives.

2. Lifelong Learning

- Cognitive exercise keeps neural wiring sharp.
- Reading, puzzles, and new skills delay decline.

3. Positive Outlook

- Optimism correlates with reduced disease risk and longer life.
- Gratitude practices "rewire" mental software.

Preventive Maintenance Habits

1. Routine Check-Ups

- Annual physical exams, blood tests.
- Dental care every 6 months.
- Age-appropriate screenings (colon, prostate, breast, bone density).

2. Early Detection

Catching problems early = simpler fixes. Preventive care is like an oil change — far cheaper than replacing the engine.

Troubleshooting Lifestyle Errors

- **Skipping sleep:** Leads to faster cognitive decline, immune weakness.
- **Chronic stress:** Accelerates cardiovascular breakdown.
- **Smoking/vaping:** Corrodes respiratory and vascular systems.
- **Excessive alcohol:** Weakens liver, brain, and heart.
- **Poor posture/inactivity:** Creates joint dysfunction and chronic pain.

Like poor fuel in a car, these habits slowly but surely clog your system.

Operating Tips for Longevity

1. **Move daily, in big and small ways.**
2. **Eat mostly whole, nutrient-dense foods.**
3. **Hydrate consistently.**
4. **Protect sleep as sacred.**
5. **Balance stress with calm practices.**
6. **Build strong social bonds.**
7. **Get regular check-ups.**
8. **Stay curious and keep learning.**
9. **Avoid corrosive habits (smoking, excess alcohol).**

Longevity isn't luck — it's **engineering plus maintenance**. The human body is built with incredible resilience, but every decision either adds miles to your healthspan or wears the system down prematurely.

By tuning fuel, movement, recovery, mindset, and environment, you give your machine not just longer life, but better life. A finely tuned system doesn't just survive decades — it thrives through them.

Chapter 19

Performance Tracking: Metrics That Matter

Gauges and Dashboards

Every advanced machine comes with gauges: fuel levels, RPM, oil pressure, tire sensors. Pilots monitor dozens of dials during flight. Mechanics rely on diagnostic readouts to tune performance.

Your body also provides **metrics** — both measurable data (heart rate, blood pressure, body composition) and subjective feedback (energy levels, mood, performance). These gauges help you monitor health, track progress, and detect problems before they escalate.

This chapter explores the key metrics worth monitoring, how often to check them, and how to interpret them for long-term optimization.

The Role of Tracking

1. Feedback Loop

- Data tells you if habits are working.
- Numbers highlight trends you might miss in daily fluctuations.

2. Motivation & Accountability

- Tracking builds consistency.
- Progress charts reinforce positive behavior.

3. Early Detection

- Rising blood pressure, falling sleep quality, or declining strength are early warning lights.

Daily Metrics

1. Resting Heart Rate (RHR)

- **Normal:** 60–100 bpm; athletes 30–50.
- **Why it matters:** Lower RHR = more efficient heart.
- **Tracking:** Morning pulse check or wearable device. Rising trend = fatigue, illness, overtraining.

2. Sleep

- **Metrics:** Total hours, quality (deep/REM stages), consistency.
- **Why it matters:** Sleep regulates recovery, hormones, mood.
- **Tools:** Sleep diary, wearables, apps.

3. Energy & Mood

- **Subjective scale:** Rate 1–10 daily.
- **Why it matters:** Captures stress load, recovery, and mental health.

4. Nutrition & Hydration

- **Track:** Food quality, water intake.
- **Why it matters:** Fuel consistency = stable performance.

Weekly Metrics

1. Training Volume

- Sets, reps, mileage, minutes of activity.
- Prevents overtraining and ensures progressive overload.

2. Body Weight & Circumference

- Track weekly, not daily (to avoid noise).
- Waist circumference is a strong predictor of metabolic health.

3. Strength Benchmarks

- Reps, loads, or time-to-fatigue.
- Ensure slow, steady progress over weeks.

4. Mobility Checks

- Can you touch your toes?
- Can you squat comfortably?
- Track movement quality as much as numbers.

Monthly Metrics

1. Body Composition

- Muscle vs. fat, not just total weight.

- Tools: Skinfold calipers, DEXA scans, smart scales (with caution).

2. Resting Heart Rate Trends

- Look at long-term patterns.
- A 5–10 bpm increase = possible overtraining, stress, or illness.

3. Blood Pressure (home check)

- Ideal: ~120/80 mmHg.
- Persistent >140/90 = see professional.

4. Recovery Indicators

- Track soreness, fatigue, and motivation monthly.

Annual Metrics

1. Medical Exams

- Full check-up: blood tests, cholesterol, blood sugar, vitamin levels.
- Update baseline each year.

2. Fitness Tests

- **VO$_2$ max:** Cardiovascular efficiency.

- **Strength tests:** 1-rep max or endurance versions.
- **Mobility tests:** Functional movement screen.

3. Dental & Vision

- Routine checks are part of system health.

4. Mental Health Check-In

- Assess stress, life satisfaction, mood patterns.

How to Interpret Metrics

1. Look for Trends, Not Single Points

- One bad night of sleep ≠ problem.
- Months of poor sleep = warning.

2. Understand Context

- Elevated heart rate after illness = normal.
- Elevated heart rate for weeks = issue.

3. Balance Objective & Subjective Data

- Numbers matter but so does "how you feel."
- If data looks fine but you feel off, trust your instincts.

Tools for Tracking

- **Wearables:** Smartwatches, fitness trackers.
- **Apps:** Nutrition logs, sleep trackers, training logs.
- **Manual logs:** Journals or spreadsheets for personal trends.
- **Professional tests:** Bloodwork, scans, and lab assessments.

Tip: Choose tools you'll actually use. Consistency beats complexity.

Common Mistakes in Tracking

- **Tracking too much.** Overload of data leads to analysis paralysis.
- **Ignoring patterns.** Numbers without reflection = wasted effort.
- **Comparing to others.** Your metrics = your machine, not someone else's.
- **Chasing vanity metrics.** Weight alone ≠ health.

Operating Tips for Tracking

1. **Pick 3–5 core metrics** to track consistently.
2. **Review weekly.** Spot trends early.
3. **Keep it simple.** Tools only matter if you use them.
4. **Track objectively and subjectively.** Balance numbers with feelings.
5. **Act on the data.** If something's off, adjust fuel, recovery, or training.

Machines run best when operators monitor gauges, catch small deviations early, and act before breakdowns occur. Your body works the same way. Tracking isn't about perfection or obsession — it's about awareness, progress, and preventive maintenance.

By learning which metrics matter and paying attention to trends, you become a skilled operator of your machine, keeping it tuned for decades of reliable performance.

Chapter 20

Extending the Warranty: Preventive Care & Medical Advances

Keeping the Machine Covered

Every machine comes with a warranty — a guarantee of function for a certain time if properly maintained. With cars, warranties extend if you follow the service schedule. With electronics, extended plans cover repairs or replacements.

The human body doesn't come with paperwork, but it does come with **a built-in service warranty**: the capacity for decades of reliable function, provided you invest in preventive care. And now, thanks to medical advances, we can extend that warranty further than ever before.

This chapter explores how preventive medicine, screenings, and emerging technologies can help you keep your machine performing at its best for as long as possible.

The Philosophy of Preventive Care

1. Prevention Beats Repair

- Fixing a problem after it breaks is always harder, costlier, and riskier.
- Preventive care finds small issues early, when they are easiest to repair.

2. Warranty Coverage = Lifestyle + Medicine

- Daily habits are your first line of coverage.

- Preventive healthcare expands the warranty by detecting silent issues (high blood pressure, cholesterol, diabetes) before symptoms appear.

The Core Preventive Checks

1. Annual Physical Exam

- Comprehensive assessment of vitals, weight, blood pressure, heart and lung sounds.
- Provides baseline data to compare year after year.

2. Blood Tests

- **Basic metabolic panel:** Glucose, electrolytes, kidney function.
- **Lipid panel:** Cholesterol and triglycerides.
- **Complete blood count:** Detects anemia, infection, immune status.
- **Hormone checks:** Thyroid, testosterone, estrogen, cortisol if symptomatic.

3. Cancer Screenings

- **Colonoscopy:** Starting around age 45–50.
- **Mammograms:** For women, typically 40+.
- **Prostate checks:** For men, typically 50+.
- **Skin checks:** Regular dermatology exams for new or changing moles.

4. Dental & Vision

- Dental visits every 6 months. Oral health strongly links to heart health.
- Eye exams every 1–2 years; more frequent if vision changes or conditions like diabetes are present.

Early Detection Technologies

Modern medicine offers **new diagnostic tools** that detect problems earlier than ever:

- **CT calcium scoring:** Measures plaque buildup in heart arteries.
- **DEXA scans:** Assess bone density to predict fracture risk.
- **Continuous glucose monitors (CGM):** Real-time feedback on blood sugar response.
- **Wearables:** Track heart rate variability, oxygen levels, sleep cycles.
- **Genetic testing:** Identifies predispositions for diseases like Alzheimer's, heart disease, or cancer.

These are like adding extra sensors to your car's dashboard — giving more detailed data before something goes wrong.

Medical Advances Extending the Warranty

1. Regenerative Medicine

- Stem cell therapies and tissue engineering aim to repair or replace damaged tissues.
- Early uses: cartilage repair, tendon healing.

2. Personalized Medicine

- Treatments tailored to your genetic profile.
- Optimized drug dosing, targeted cancer therapies.

3. Longevity Science

- Research on calorie restriction mimetics, senolytics (removing "zombie" cells), and anti-aging compounds.
- Still emerging but promising for extending healthspan.

4. Surgical & Device Advances

- Minimally invasive surgeries = faster recovery.
- Artificial joints, pacemakers, and stents extend quality of life.

Your Role in Warranty Extension

Medical advances help, but you remain the **primary operator** of your machine.

- **Follow service schedule:** Routine exams, screenings, vaccinations.
- **Report dashboard lights:** Don't ignore new symptoms.
- **Maintain daily habits:** Sleep, fuel, exercise, stress balance.
- **Stay informed:** Health knowledge evolves; adapt your practices.

Common Mistakes in Preventive Care

- **Only going to the doctor when sick.** Prevention = early detection.
- **Skipping screenings.** Many diseases are silent until advanced.
- **Neglecting dental/vision.** These are early windows into systemic health.
- **Relying only on technology.** Gadgets help, but daily habits remain foundational.

Operating Tips for Extending the Warranty

1. **Book annual check-ups.** Don't skip them.
2. **Know your numbers.** Blood pressure, cholesterol, glucose, BMI.
3. **Leverage technology.** Use wearables and apps to monitor health.
4. **Consider early screenings.** Especially if family history raises risk.
5. **Stay proactive, not reactive.** Prevention is always cheaper than repair.

Machines last longer when cared for, inspected, and upgraded. The human body is no exception. With modern preventive medicine, regular check-ups, and emerging medical advances, your body's **warranty can be extended decades beyond what was once possible.**

Your role is simple but powerful: adopt lifestyle habits from earlier chapters, use preventive healthcare as your inspection system, and take advantage of modern advances. The result is not just longer life — it's a longer **healthspan**, where your machine performs beautifully year after year.

Part 6

Beyond Standard Use

Chapter 21

Operating in Extreme Conditions

Pushing the Machine Beyond Standard Specs

Every machine has a normal operating range — safe temperature zones, pressure limits, altitude ceilings. Exceed those parameters, and performance changes. Sometimes systems adapt, sometimes they fail.

The human body is remarkably adaptable. It can function in deserts, mountaintops, arctic tundra, and deep water. But in each environment, stress on the system increases, requiring different strategies for survival and performance.

This chapter explains how your body operates under **extreme conditions** and how to prepare, protect, and adapt when you push beyond everyday limits.

Heat: High-Temperature Stress

1. How the Body Cools

- **Sweating:** Evaporation releases heat (up to 2 liters/hour in intense heat).
- **Vasodilation:** Blood vessels widen to bring heat to the skin.
- **Increased heart rate:** Circulatory system works harder to move blood to the surface.

2. Performance Effects

- Dehydration reduces blood volume.
- Heart must pump harder, reducing endurance.
- Risk of cramps, heat exhaustion, heat stroke.

3. Troubleshooting in Heat

- **Hydration:** Replace water and electrolytes.

- **Acclimatization:** Body adapts in ~7–14 days with earlier sweating and better cooling.
- **Clothing:** Light, breathable fabrics enhance evaporation.
- **Warning lights:** Dizziness, confusion, cessation of sweating = danger zone.

Cold: Low-Temperature Stress

1. How the Body Warms

- **Vasoconstriction:** Blood vessels narrow to preserve core temperature.
- **Shivering:** Muscle activity generates heat.
- **Brown fat activation:** In infants and some adults, burns calories for heat.

2. Performance Effects

- Muscles stiffen, reducing power and agility.
- Fine motor control decreases.
- Risk of frostbite and hypothermia.

3. Troubleshooting in Cold

- **Layering:** Trap heat while wicking sweat away.
- **Fueling:** Higher calorie needs (shivering burns energy).
- **Movement:** Keep moving to maintain heat.

- **Warning lights:** Numbness, slurred speech, confusion, uncontrolled shivering.

Altitude: Thin-Air Stress

1. What Changes at Altitude

- Less oxygen per breath.
- Reduced endurance and mental clarity.
- Body compensates with faster breathing and increased heart rate.

2. Adaptations

- Kidneys excrete bicarbonate to balance blood pH.
- Over days, body produces more red blood cells to carry oxygen.
- Long-term acclimatization enhances endurance at sea level.

3. Troubleshooting in Altitude

- **Acclimate slowly:** Ascend gradually; "climb high, sleep low."
- **Hydrate more:** Dry air increases water loss.
- **Fuel on carbs:** Oxygen-efficient fuel at altitude.
- **Warning lights:** Headache, nausea, confusion = altitude sickness (descend immediately if severe).

Underwater: Pressure Stress

1. Effects of Pressure

- Every 10 meters (~33 feet) depth = pressure increases by 1 atmosphere.
- Air spaces compress (lungs, ears, sinuses).
- Breathing dense air increases effort.

2. Adaptations

- Diving reflex: Slowed heart rate, blood shift to protect organs.
- Oxygen conservation mechanisms kick in.

3. Troubleshooting Underwater

- **Equalization:** Release ear/sinus pressure regularly.
- **Slow ascent:** Prevents decompression sickness ("the bends").
- **Equipment reliance:** SCUBA extends limits but requires precision.
- **Warning lights:** Dizziness, disorientation, joint pain post-dive = possible decompression sickness.

Extreme Effort & Stress

Not all extremes are environmental — some are situational.

1. High-Intensity Effort

- Sprinting, heavy lifting push cardiovascular and muscular systems to limits.
- Lactic acid buildup causes temporary fatigue.
- Adaptation = stronger, faster systems with recovery.

2. Psychological Stress

- Fight-or-flight activates adrenaline and cortisol.
- Short bursts enhance survival; chronic overload damages the system.
- Mental resilience training is as important as physical.

Common Mistakes in Extreme Conditions

- **Overconfidence:** Assuming your machine works the same in all environments.
- **Ignoring warning lights:** Heat stroke, frostbite, altitude sickness escalate quickly.

- **Underestimating hydration/fuel needs:** Extremes double energy and water demands.
- **Skipping acclimatization:** Body needs time to adjust.

Operating Tips for Extremes

1. **Respect the limits.** The machine adapts, but only gradually.
2. **Acclimate properly.** Don't rush heat, cold, or altitude adaptation.
3. **Fuel and hydrate more.** Demands increase under stress.
4. **Dress and gear smart.** Protect skin, joints, lungs in harsh environments.
5. **Monitor dashboard lights.** Confusion, dizziness, or uncontrolled shivering = stop.
6. **Train resilience.** Cold showers, heat exposure, or altitude training can prep systems.

Your body is a masterpiece of engineering — capable of operating across deserts, mountains, oceans, and arctic landscapes. No other machine comes close to this adaptability. But even advanced systems have limits.

By respecting the operating range, preparing intelligently, and learning the warning signs, you can push your machine beyond standard specs safely and effectively.

Chapter 22

Warranty & Service Life

The Original Warranty

Every machine is designed with an expected service life. Cars have mileage estimates, aircraft have flight-hour limits, and electronics come with expiration dates.

Your body, too, has a **built-in warranty**. Barring accident or disease, the human body is engineered to last **70–90 years**, with the potential for many more. But how much of that time is spent in good working order — your **healthspan** — depends on how you operate and maintain your system.

This chapter explores how lifestyle, environment, and preventive care determine whether you maximize the full warranty or cut your service life short.

Design of the Human Machine

1. Genetic Blueprint

- Genes set baseline durability: some people are naturally more resilient.
- But **lifestyle factors account for ~70%** of longevity differences.

2. Built-In Redundancy

- Two kidneys, two lungs, backup circulation routes.
- Body compensates for damage surprisingly well — until reserves run out.

3. Expected Range

- Average life expectancy: ~76–80 in many developed nations.
- Maximum recorded lifespan: 122 years.

- Most failures come not from design flaws but from misuse, neglect, or breakdowns preventable with maintenance.

What Shortens Service Life

1. Corrosive Fuels

- Smoking, excess alcohol, ultra-processed foods accelerate decay.
- Like poor-quality fuel in an engine, they clog, corrode, and wear systems prematurely.

2. Overload Stress

- Chronic stress = constant high RPMs.
- Leads to cardiovascular wear, immune suppression, mental burnout.

3. Sedentary Living

- Inactivity weakens the frame, circulation, and power supply.
- Sitting long-term is like letting a machine idle endlessly — parts seize up.

4. Ignored Warning Lights

- Small issues left unchecked (high blood pressure, pain, fatigue) often lead to major breakdowns.

What Extends Service Life

1. Preventive Maintenance

- Annual check-ups and screenings = catching issues early.

2. Quality Fuel

- Balanced, whole-food nutrition keeps systems clean and efficient.

3. Movement

- Strength training preserves muscle and bone.
- Cardio sustains circulation.
- Mobility preserves freedom of movement.

4. Stress Balance

- Downtime, recovery, and mental health care reduce "wear and tear."

5. Social & Mental Factors

- Strong relationships, purpose, and optimism extend healthspan.
- Mental health is as protective as physical maintenance.

Service by the Decade

20s–30s: Installation & Optimization

- Peak performance years.
- Build habits — fitness, nutrition, recovery — that pay off for decades.

40s–50s: Wear Management

- Subtle declines begin.
- Prioritize strength and preventive care. Screen for silent issues.

60s–70s: Preservation

- Focus shifts to independence, stability, and cognitive health.
- Longevity = mobility + mental sharpness.

80s and Beyond: Resilience

- Machines with proper maintenance still run well.
- Social connection, daily movement, and medical support sustain quality of life.

The Balance of Healthspan vs. Lifespan

1. Long Life vs. Good Life

- Living longer doesn't matter if the last 20 years are spent immobile, in pain, or dependent.
- Goal: Extend **healthspan** so your best years stretch far into older age.

2. Compression of Morbidity

- Ideal scenario: long life with minimal sickness at the very end.
- Achieved through decades of balanced maintenance.

Legacy of a Well-Maintained Machine

1. Independence

- Maintaining muscle, balance, and mental sharpness preserves freedom.

2. Energy

- Even at older ages, vitality fuels work, hobbies, family, and joy.

3. Example

- A well-maintained body inspires future generations to value theirs.

Operating Tips for Maximizing Warranty

1. **Respect daily maintenance.** Small habits extend lifespan.
2. **Keep up service checks.** Screenings, blood work, and exams catch early issues.
3. **Balance performance with preservation.** Push limits but also recover.
4. **Avoid corrosive fuels.** Smoking, excess alcohol, and junk food shorten service life.

5. **Stay connected.** Relationships, purpose, and joy protect long-term health.
6. **Remember: healthspan > lifespan.** Quality of life matters more than just years.

Your body is the most advanced piece of engineering you'll ever own. It comes with a remarkable service life — decades of reliable, adaptable function. But whether you get the full warranty or face early breakdown depends largely on **how you operate the machine**.

With the right fuel, movement, recovery, preventive checks, and mindset, you can maximize both lifespan and healthspan — ensuring that when the final shutdown eventually comes, it happens after a long, fulfilling, high-performance journey.

Epilogue

The Operator's Responsibility

Every machine has a manual, but most people skim it or never open it at all. They rely on trial and error, assuming the system will just work — until it doesn't.

The difference between machines and the human body is that you only get one. No replacements, no trade-ins, no extended warranty beyond what you create for yourself.

You now hold what many never receive: a guide to understanding, operating, maintaining, and optimizing the most advanced piece of engineering on the planet.

The Masterpiece You Operate

Your body is a **supercomputer, a high-performance vehicle, and a resilient survival system all in one**.

- It repairs itself.
- It adapts to new environments.
- It learns and rewires.
- It sustains decades of performance with the right care.

No engineered device comes close. Even the most advanced machines break down within years. But your system, if properly cared for, is designed to function for decades — sometimes more than a century.

The Operator's Choice

Every day, you make small decisions that either:

- **Preserve and optimize** your system, or
- **Degrade and shorten** its performance.

Fuel, movement, recovery, mindset, environment — these are levers you can adjust. Ignore them, and the system runs down. Respect them, and the system thrives.

It's not about perfection. It's about awareness. About becoming an intentional operator rather than a passive one.

The Legacy of Maintenance

How you run your machine doesn't just affect you. It affects everyone around you:

- Your energy fuels your work, family, and relationships.
- Your health preserves independence, reducing burden on others.
- Your habits create examples — for children, peers, and communities.

A well-maintained human body isn't just a personal asset. It's a social contribution.

Your Next Steps

This manual is not meant to be read once and shelved. It's a reference, a reminder, a roadmap. The real work happens in the small choices after you close this book:

- Choosing water instead of soda.
- Taking a walk instead of scrolling.
- Going to bed instead of watching "one more episode."
- Scheduling the check-up instead of postponing it again.

The manual provides the knowledge. **You provide the discipline and consistency.**

From Operator to Master

You were born with the most extraordinary machine ever built. Most people never read the instructions. But you now have the tools to:

- Prevent breakdowns.
- Optimize performance.
- Extend the warranty.
- Enjoy decades of reliable, vibrant function.

Your body is not disposable. It's not replaceable. It's the one piece of equipment you'll own for life.

Operate it with respect, with curiosity, and with care — and it will reward you with strength, clarity, and longevity beyond what most imagine possible.

This is your user manual. But the responsibility is yours.

Bibliography

Anatomy & Physiology

- American College of Sports Medicine. *ACSM's Guidelines for Exercise Testing and Prescription.* 11th ed. Philadelphia: Wolters Kluwer, 2021.
- Hall, John E., and Michael E. Hall. *Guyton and Hall Textbook of Medical Physiology.* 14th ed. Philadelphia: Elsevier, 2020.
- Martini, Frederic H., Judi L. Nath, and Edwin F. Bartholomew. *Fundamentals of Anatomy & Physiology.* 12th ed. New York: Pearson, 2020.
- Tortora, Gerard J., and Bryan Derrickson. *Principles of Anatomy and Physiology.* 16th ed. Hoboken, NJ: Wiley, 2021.

Biomechanics & Movement

- McGinnis, Peter M. *Biomechanics of Sport and Exercise.* 4th ed. Champaign, IL: Human Kinetics, 2020.
- Neumann, Donald A. *Kinesiology of the Musculoskeletal System: Foundations for Rehabilitation.* 3rd ed. St. Louis, MO: Elsevier, 2017.
- Zatsiorsky, Vladimir M., and William J. Kraemer. *Science and Practice of Strength Training.* 2nd ed. Champaign, IL: Human Kinetics, 2006.

Exercise Science & Training

- Baechle, Thomas R., and Roger W. Earle. *Essentials of Strength Training and Conditioning.* 4th ed. Champaign, IL: Human Kinetics, 2015.
- McArdle, William D., Frank I. Katch, and Victor L. Katch. *Exercise Physiology: Nutrition, Energy, and Human Performance.* 10th ed. Philadelphia: Wolters Kluwer, 2022.
- Schoenfeld, Brad J. *Science and Development of Muscle Hypertrophy.* 2nd ed. Champaign, IL: Human Kinetics, 2020.

Nutrition & Health

- Campbell, T. Colin, and Thomas M. Campbell. *The China Study: The Most Comprehensive Study of Nutrition Ever Conducted.* Dallas: BenBella Books, 2006.
- Gropper, Sareen S., and Jack L. Smith. *Advanced Nutrition and Human Metabolism.* 8th ed. Boston: Cengage Learning, 2020.
- Willett, Walter C., and Patrick J. Skerrett. *Eat, Drink, and Be Healthy: The Harvard Medical School Guide to Healthy Eating.* New York: Free Press, 2017.

Sleep, Stress, and Recovery

- McEwen, Bruce S. *The End of Stress as We Know It.* Washington, DC: Dana Press, 2002.
- Selye, Hans. *The Stress of Life.* New York: McGraw-Hill, 1956.
- Walker, Matthew. *Why We Sleep: Unlocking the Power of Sleep and Dreams.* New York: Scribner, 2017.

Preventive Medicine & Longevity

- Buettner, Dan. *The Blue Zones: Lessons for Living Longer from the People Who've Lived the Longest.* Washington, DC: National Geographic, 2012.
- DeMaria, Anthony N., et al. "Cardiovascular Disease Prevention: Lifestyle and Risk Factor Management." *Journal of the American College of Cardiology* 72, no. 14 (2018): 1760–73.
- Fontana, Luigi, et al. "Extending Healthy Life Span—From Yeast to Humans." *Science* 328, no. 5976 (2010): 321–26.

Mental & Emotional Health

- Kabat-Zinn, Jon. *Full Catastrophe Living: Using the Wisdom of Your Body and Mind to Face Stress, Pain, and Illness.* New York: Bantam Books, 2013.
- Ratey, John J. *Spark: The Revolutionary New Science of Exercise and the Brain.* New York: Little, Brown Spark, 2008.
- Sapolsky, Robert M. *Why Zebras Don't Get Ulcers.* 3rd ed. New York: Holt Paperbacks, 2004.

General Audience Science & Inspiration

- Bryson, Bill. *The Body: A Guide for Occupants.* New York: Doubleday, 2019.
- Greger, Michael, M.D., and Gene Stone. *How Not to Die.* New York: Flatiron Books, 2015.
- Howard, Pierce J. *The Owner's Manual for the Brain.* 4th ed. New York: HarperCollins, 2014.

www.ingramcontent.com/pod-product-compliance
Lightning Source LLC
Chambersburg PA
CBHW060456030426
42337CB00015B/1612